T0261204

RETHINKING PROFESSIONAL GOVERNANCE

International directions in healthcare

Edited by Ellen Kuhlmann and Mike Saks

First published in Great Britain in 2008 by

The Policy Press
University of Bristol
Fourth Floor
Beacon House
Queen's Road
Bristol BS8 1QU
UK

Tel +44 (0)117 331 4054
Fax +44 (0)117 331 4093
e-mail tpp-info@bristol.ac.uk
www.policypress.org.uk

British Library Cataloguing in Publication Data
A catalogue record for this book is available from the British Library.

Library of Congress Cataloging-in-Publication Data
A catalog record for this book has been requested.

ISBN 978 1 86134 956 9 hardcover

Cover design by Qube Design.
Front cover: photograph kindly supplied by Paul Green.

Contents

List of tables and figures

Tables

Figures

Notes on contributors

Judith Allsop is Professor of Health Policy at the University of Lincoln, UK and Professor emerita of London South Bank University, UK.
Email: jallsop@lincoln.ac.uk

Ivy Lynn Bourgeault is Associate Professor in the Department of Health, Aging and Society/Sociology at McMaster University, Canada, and Canada Research Chair in Comparative Health Labour Policy.
Email: bourgea@mcmaster.ca

Rosalie A. Boyce is Visiting Research Advisor at the School of Pharmacy, University of Queensland, Brisbane, Australia.
Email: r.boyce@uq.edu.au

Viola Burau is Associate Professor in Public Policy in the Department of Political Science, University of Aarhus, Denmark.
Email: viola@ps.au.dk

Michael Calnan is Professor of Medical Sociology at the School of Social Policy, Sociology and Social Research, University of Kent, UK.
Email: m.w.calnan@kent.ac.uk

Rannveig Dahle is Senior Researcher at Norwegian Social Research, NOVA, Oslo, Norway.
Email: rannveig.dahle@nova.no

Elizabeth Darling is a Registered Midwife and MSc graduate of the Department of Clinical Epidemiology and Biostatistics, McMaster University, Canada.
Email: ldarling@idirect.com

Katalin Formadi is Lecturer in the Tourism Department, University of Pannonia, Veszprém and PhD student at the University of Corvinus, Budapest, Hungary.
Email: formadi@turizmus.vein.hu

Elena Iarskaia-Smirnova is Professor of Sociology in the Department of Social Anthropology and Social Work, Saratov State Technical University, Russia.
Email: iarskaia@jsps.ru

Kathryn Jones is Senior Research Fellow in the Department of Public Policy, De Montfort University, Leicester, UK.
Email: kljones@dmu.ac.uk

Ellen Kuhlmann is Senior Lecturer in the Department of Social and Policy Sciences, University of Bath, UK.
Email: e.c.kuhlmann@bath.ac.uk

Aurelija Novelskaite is Researcher at the Institute for Social Research in Vilnius, and Lecturer at the Faculty of Humanities, Vilnius University Kaunas, Lithuania.
Email: novelskaite@ktl.mii.lt

Majda Pahor is Associate Professor of Sociology of Health and Illness at the School of Health Studies, University of Ljubljana, Slovenia.
Email: majda.pahor@vsz.uni-lj.si

Joana Sousa Ribeiro is a PhD student in Sociology at the Economic School and Associate Researcher at the Centre for Social Studies, University of Coimbra, Portugal.
Email: joanaribeiro@ces.uc.pt

Elianne Riska is Professor of Sociology at the Swedish School of Social Sciences, University of Helsinki, Finland.
Email: elianne.riska@helsinki.fi

Pavel Romanov is Professor of Sociology in the Department of Social Anthropology and Social Work and Director of the Centre for Social Policy and Gender Studies, Saratov State Technical University, Russia.
Email: romanov@jsps.ru

Rosemary Rowe is Service Improvement Manager at the Bath & North East Somerset Primary Care Trust, Bath, UK.
Email: rosie.rowe@banes-pct.nhs.uk

Mike Saks is Pro Vice Chancellor and Professor of Health and Community Studies at the University of Lincoln, UK.
Email: msaks@lincoln.ac.uk

Gry Skogheim is Lecturer in the Department of Health Education, University College Tromsø, Norway.
Email: Gry.Skogheim@hitos.no

Karsten Vrangbæk is Associate Professor in the Department of Political Science, University of Copenhagen, Denmark.
Email: kv@ifs.ku.dk.

Sirpa Wrede is Academy Research Fellow of the Academy of Finland and Researcher at the Swedish School of Social Sciences, University of Helsinki, Finland.
Email: sirpa.wrede@helsinki.fi

Changing patterns of health professional governance

Ellen Kuhlmann and Mike Saks

Across many countries professional governance is under the spotlight of health policy makers and subject to public debate. This book provides new data and geopolitical perspectives in the debate over how to govern healthcare. It sets out to highlight new international directions and the significance of national contexts for the changing health workforce based on complex sets of cultural and institutional regulatory patterns. One central goal of the new health policies that are emerging is accountability and control of professionals, which in turn calls for tighter regulation and new forms of professional development. However, the dominant models of health reform have been developed in Anglo–American health systems and need broader comparative analysis and new approaches.

One novel feature of the book is the linkage of international directions in professional governance and workforce change to developments in the various continental European countries, including the different types of transformation states of Southern, Central and Eastern Europe. Another novelty is the expansion of the public debate on professional governance – hitherto mainly limited to physicians and medical self-regulation – to a broad range of healthcare providers, from nurses and midwives to alternative therapists and health support workers. A third innovative feature is the framing of professional development in the context of broader societal trends involving increasing flexibility, mobility and individualisation as well as changing gender arrangements and ethnic diversity. The connecting link between the different topics and countries is the exploration of political, institutional and cultural changes – related to globalisation, European unification and new governance approaches – and workforce dynamics.

In bringing together research from a wide range of continental European countries – as well as the United Kingdom (UK), Canada and Australia – the book therefore highlights different arenas of governance and the various players involved in the policy process. It helps to clarify the significance of national regulatory frameworks and better understand the enabling conditions for, and the barriers to, making professionals more accountable to a more demanding public. As such, it opens up new perspectives on the policy options to ensure that public services and the groups that deliver these are more responsive to the interests of citizens.

The changing context of professional governance

In terms of the changing context, professional governance faces a number of new challenges arising from economic constraints, developing medical technologies and an increase in chronic illnesses, as well as new modes of social citizenship. Across countries, tighter regulation of healthcare providers together with improved participation of service users and considerations of the safety of the public has increased the accountability of professionals. This has enhanced the shift from a supply-led to a more demand-led organisation and delivery of healthcare services. The pressures for change and the models for reform have been discussed extensively in research on health policy (see, for example, Allsop and Saks, 2002; Maynard and Street, 2006; Blank and Burau, 2007). Our attention now shifts to the different areas of governance and how they are connected with professional development and workforce change.

Existing research suggests that there has been a specific move towards more inclusive and collaborative forms of governing healthcare providers, such as network-based and partnership governance, and a general shift towards hybrid forms of governance (Dent, 2003; Blank and Burau, 2004). New models of governance are based on meso-level governing practices through a number of performance measurements, such as clinical guidelines, quality reports, benchmarks and other forms of assessment (Gray and Harrison, 2004). While the 'remaking' of governance (Newman, 2005) applies to the entire service sector, in healthcare the transformations are linked to specific configurations of state–professions and professions–citizens relationships. These are centred on the medical model of self-regulation, based on public trust in professionals to act in the interests of citizens. In addition, Europeanisation and globalisation may challenge the national 'healthcare state' (Moran, 1999) and bring new uncertainties to the health policy process, although healthcare fundamentally remains a matter of national regulation (Mossialos and McKee, 2002).

Changes in governance and the interplay of different arrangements for governance call for new approaches to researching healthcare (Saks and Allsop, 2007). Existing typologies used for the comparison of healthcare systems do not adequately reflect the changes currently under way. In particular, they are biased towards medical care and doctors, and may not therefore be appropriate when it comes to the assessment of a wide range of health professional groups, still less meso-level governance practices (Burau and Blank, 2006; Wrede et al, 2006). New theoretical approaches and in-depth research that moves beyond medical governance and macro-level analysis of data are therefore needed to examine the changing international governance of healthcare.

Researching the changing international governance in healthcare

This edited collection responds to the new demands for research on changing international governance in various ways. One central strength of the volume is the linkage made between policy and workforce change. An approach to governance as different sets of practices and regulatory mechanisms (Newman, 2005) provides the connecting link between changing policies and changing professions. Studying new forms of governance at the interface of policy and professions takes account of the diversity of interests and players involved in the translation of new policies into practice. This approach may contribute to a wider debate on policy learning and public accountability: it helps to explore how 'social policy as a productive force' (Room, 2007, p 241) intersects with driving forces from within the professions and society at large. To this end, perspectives on the sociology of professions provide deeper insights into the state–professions relationship and the tensions between the professional and public interest (see, for instance, Johnson et al, 1995; Saks and Kuhlmann, 2006).

Another strength of the book is its focus on the combination of comparative analysis, case studies in countries with different health systems and in-depth research on a range of professional groups and regulatory mechanisms. The studies presented here cover a wide range of societies encompassing many varieties of changing health and welfare systems, which include the three classic types of welfare state provision of healthcare by national health services in Anglo-Saxon countries, different models of welfare regulation in the Nordic countries and corporatist-oriented systems of social health insurance. This is complemented by a discussion of the developing and mixed health systems in the south, middle and east of Europe.

One important criterion for the selection of countries was to ensure that there is a sufficient diversity of models of 'public responsibility' for the provision of healthcare and pathways to modernisation in the general retrenchment of welfare state services. With respect to transformations in European welfare state systems, Room (2007, p 240) argues that the differences between Anglo-Saxon and Scandinavian models – both representing successful socioeconomic development – and the situation in continental European countries are crucial to cross-national policy learning, which also means 'that piecemeal adaptation of "best practices" from the front-runners may merely exacerbate problems'. The challenges of a 'globalised recipe' for reform may be even greater when it comes to the governance of health professions, given the dominance of the nation state in this area of welfare state transformations (Mossialos and McKee, 2002). To this end, the 'Westernisation' of Central and Eastern European countries with the introduction of markets in historically developed frameworks of state responsibility – based on Soviet bureaucracy and socialist values – provide particularly interesting contexts for exploring governance.

Following the criticism of comparisons that reduce health policy to health systems (Blank and Burau, 2004) – or, more generally, the processes of 'infantalisation' that subordinate social policy to wider trends (Clarke, 2004, p 3) – the book examines major questions and challenges raised by changing patterns of professional governance across countries rather than assuming the uniform and linear impact of policies in this area. While individual chapters do not provide systematic international comparisons, the collection of chapters provides deep insights into the connectivity of policy and workforce dynamics and how they play out in a range of specific national contexts. As such, the text adds further theoretical and geopolitical perspectives to the debate on changing governance in healthcare – as well as providing new empirical data for analysing this field.

New health policies: remaking state–professions–citizens relationships

Internationally, new health policies generally aim to provide increased efficiency in the provision and delivery of services and greater responsiveness to user demands. This has been achieved mainly through the introduction of internal markets and managerialist regimes together with improved user participation and broadening the scope of stakeholders and interests involved in the policy process. As such, decentralisation, contractualisation and the competition of providers are key elements of new health policies and incentive structures. Various studies have highlighted the new forms of political power embedded in changing governance practices and public sector reform and the 'instabilities and contradictions that may be produced in the process of reform' (Newman, 2005, p 7). Focusing on these power relations and tensions also helps us to explore changes in the configuration of state–professions and professions–citizens relationships in healthcare.

New health policies frequently challenge existing power structures, not least medical self-regulation and trust in the altruistic mission of professionalism (see, for instance, DH, 2006, 2007). Controversy remains, however, as to whether they actually shift the balance of power and their effects on the provision of healthcare. While some authors emphasise the challenges of marketisation and managerialism (as, for example, Hunter, 2006), others are more sceptical about the fall of medical 'heroism' (Davies, 2006). Yet another strand of the literature takes on the argument by Freidson (2001) that professionalism is a 'third logic' and underscores the benefits of professionalism, for instance by assuring trust in public services and reducing the costs of governmental action and control (Duyvendak et al, 2006; Evetts, 2006).

Existing research also brings into view a number of issues – including the potentially adverse effects of new health policies. 'Old power structures' (Salter, 2002) may not be overcome as easily as new policies suggest. For example, the 'micropolitics' of governance may provide new opportunities for the medical profession to assert its authority (McDonald and Harrison, 2004). Waring (2007, p 176) argues that it may well be the case that 'doctors are in fact "going through the motions" of taking up these new procedures in an effort to resist regulatory change'. Such developments have certainly been observed in the German healthcare system (Kuhlmann, 2006). However, opportunity structures are shaped by national regulatory frameworks and there may be significant national differences in policy impact on both the medical and other health professions.

Another strand of the literature focuses on the changing role of the service user and the ways in which the 'public interest' is represented in the policy process. Recent studies carried out in the UK suggest that the policy discourse of consumerism and placing 'patients first' together with change in institutional regulation may improve the inclusion of service users to some extent and in some areas, but that changes in the power structure are not necessarily sustainable (Baggott et al, 2004; Davies et al, 2006; Barnes et al, 2007; Clarke et al, 2007). Similar problems are described in the Scandinavian (Vabø, 2006) and also the German context (Kuhlmann, 2006). It is also important to note that the new agenda of 'choice' is closely linked to the various models of social citizenship and welfare state governance and may therefore be applied in different ways – even if it is increasingly relevant across 'individualised societies' and modernising welfare states (see, for instance, Hvinden and Johansson, 2007; Newman and Kuhlmann, 2007).

New health policies have important implications for the relationships between the state and the professions, and the professions and citizens. Although the shifts in the power structure may at present be weaker than assumed and adverse effects are hardly predictable, the relationships are becoming more open to change. One consequence of the move towards demand-led healthcare services is greater competition and public control of providers, thereby transforming professional self-regulation and the 'private interest government' of professions (Moran, 1999). Another consequence is that new professional groups are emerging and increasingly enter the health political stage, although often not as equal partners. This opens up a new arena in the governance of health professions, highlighting the significance of professionalisation and interprofessional relationships. Understanding such developments helps us to further explore the opportunity structures provided by new health policies and the barriers to change, especially in relation to the reconfiguration of professional boundaries.

Professional development: the reconfiguration of boundaries

New health policies can lead to new strategies on the part of health professions, which by definition are exclusionary groups. Recent increases in managerial control and the participation of service users, however, mean that the classic exclusionary tactics of the professions are no longer appropriate in healthcare. One important area where transformation can be observed 'in action' is in the establishment of more integrated and collaborative caring systems. The 'making' of a collaborative health workforce is a key element of international health policy (as highlighted by Dubois et al, 2006). The rise in long-term illnesses together with economic pressures for more effective use of human resources has created new pressures for change. It is increasingly recognised that no single profession is able to provide the care desired. There is evidence that multidisciplinary care models and teamwork approaches are more effective compared with existing models of medical care based on the fragmentation of services (see, for instance, Sicotte et al, 2002) – even though there are a number of barriers to interprofessional working.

'Tribalism' and 'boundary work' of the professions are usually perceived as the most important barriers to collaboration. This raises more general questions about how far professionalism can be transformed and the capacity – and willingness – of professions to act in the interest of citizens. A key issue is whether a new professionalism based on social inclusion is in the making, and how such a development relates to the system in which professions are embedded. Current research suggests that the willingness of professions to collaborate is significantly influenced by the organisational contexts of healthcare. A recent literature review of interprofessional relations in primary and community care, for example, showed the significance of organisational conditions for aspects of teamwork such as team structure and team processes (Xyrichis and Lowton, forthcoming). A Dutch study explored the reasons for this and compared the rationales for cooperation by providers; the authors concluded that 'policy makers must map the institutions of stakeholders and enable integrated care policy to correspond with these institutions as much as possible' (Raak et al, 2005, p 13).

The regulatory frameworks of health systems and health policy incentives seem to have an important impact on whether and how professional groups are becoming more inclusive. This highlights the significance of national contexts in exploring the options for a more collaborative health workforce (Bourgeault and Mulvale, 2006). There are considerable differences in the advancement of professionalisation among health occupational groups even within Europe, despite the fact that the Bologna agreements further the homogenisation of educational systems. National conditions also affect the regulatory structure of the health workforce. For instance, in the UK a wide range of health professional groups are now included in the newly established regulatory bodies (Allsop and Saks, 2002), while in Germany the provider side is mainly represented by the medical profession (Kuhlmann, 2006). However, there is a lack of knowledge as to whether the emergence of new professional groups and their inclusion in regulatory bodies actually changes existing patterns of professionalism and fosters more inclusive professional projects, particularly with increasing provider competition and new forms of assessment.

The reconfiguration of boundaries within and between professional groups is not only driven by new health policies and the demands of collaboration, but also a much wider picture that influences exclusionary/inclusionary practices. In this respect, for example, professional development is deeply shaped by change in gender arrangements and the sexual division of labour (see, among others, Riska, 2001; Witz and Annandale, 2006). Such workforce dynamics also arise from drivers such as new organisational models of flexible work, emerging fields of professional work 'in-between' healthcare and other sectors of the labour market, and cross-country mobility as a result of globalisation and Europeanisation (Dubois et al, 2006).

Individual mobility and the benefits derived from flexibility and the crossing of multiple boundaries in healthcare create new challenges for professions and policy makers alike in relation to the social inclusion of a diverse and fluid workforce. This requires the transformation of existing power structures – a point that is no better exemplified than in the case of marginal groups in the healthcare division of labour. In this regard, such areas as gender and ethnicity highlight the various ways in which professional boundaries both have been and can be further recast and how these are shaped by national configurations of healthcare states and cultures.

The structure of the book

This book endeavours to capture many of the key themes considered above. Centred on rethinking professional governance in the context of past, present and potential future international trends in healthcare, the volume is divided into three parts. Part One opens the book by discussing general trends and the challenges posed, and opportunities provided, by new forms of health professional governance. This is followed in Part Two by in-depth analysis of a key goal in health policy – the making of an integrated health workforce with collaborative professionals – while Part Three examines the new workforce dynamics and subsequent demands on regulation that are too often overlooked in new health policies. The main topics of workforce change and new forms of governance recur in various parts of the book and connect the chapters. These are assessed from different theoretical, methodological and geopolitical perspectives, thereby extending the 'context' of professional governance and exposing a wide range of factors to consideration.

Part One – New directions in the governance of healthcare – starts with a broad comparative approach to new international directions in the governance of healthcare, focusing on the health professions. It addresses a wide range of formal and informal regulatory mechanisms – particularly those involving the safety of patients, marketisation and managerialism, and trust relations – which are linked to national/international settings and the interest-based strategies of the professions.

Judith Allsop and Kathryn Jones focus in Chapter One on the comparative international arrangements for professional governance in medicine to protect patients, highlighting a general trend towards partnership governance. Viola Burau and Karsten Vrangbæk in Chapter Two analyse a range of country-specific pathways of re-regulation in relation to markets in healthcare, with a focus on the differences between broadly similar models of re-regulation. Moving beyond the controversies of marketisation and managerialism, Ellen Kuhlmann discusses in

Chapter Three the transformability of professional groups as mediators between the state and its citizens, using Germany as a case study. Michael Calnan and Rosemary Rowe meanwhile consider in Chapter Four how and why trust relations may be changing in the illustrative context of new forms of governance in the UK – presenting in the process a theoretical framework for explaining different forms of trust relations. Rosalie A. Boyce in Chapter Five concludes this part of the volume by examining the implications of the new public management reforms related to entrepreneurialism and managerialism for professional culture and practices in public sector health services with reference to allied health professions in Australia.

Part Two – Drivers and barriers to integration: health policies and professional development – brings into view the challenges of the new demands for social inclusion to the traditional 'boundary work' of the professions. It explores, among other things, intersections between policy and workforce change, and diverse sets of dynamics arising from organisational restructuring and the new agenda of the service user. As such, it includes an intriguing range of areas in a number of individual countries related to, but formally outside of, medicine – such as alternative medicine and midwifery.

This part of the book begins with an analysis by Ivy Lynn Bourgeault and Elizabeth Darling in Chapter Six of collaborative work and professional boundaries in maternity care, focused on Canada, where the authors explore the significance of institutional contexts that shape the opportunities for social inclusion and collaboration across macro and meso levels of governance. This leads on to a discussion by Majda Pahor in Chapter Seven of research into interprofessional relationships between nurses and doctors in Slovenia, introducing the notion of culture as a hidden organiser of professional action and identity. Sirpa Wrede in Chapter Eight then directs attention to new professional groups positioned at the bottom of the health workforce, considering the dilemmas posed by changing governance and the discourse of flexibilisation for the professional identity of auxiliary nursing in Finland. Chapter Nine by Elena Iarskaia-Smirnova and Pavel Romanov further explores the challenges of integrating emerging professional groups and the significance of culture, discussing the integration of folk medicine in healthcare in the cultural context of Russia – not least through professionalisation. Finally, Mike Saks in Chapter Ten compares the marginal, but intersecting, groups of health support workers and practitioners of complementary and alternative medicine in the UK, with particular reference to changing national policy and workforce dynamics.

Part Three – Workforce dynamics: gender, migration and mobility – shifts the focus towards the actors involved in, and the workforce dynamics surrounding, health professional governance. It discusses gender relations, along with the new and increasingly significant issues of flexible workers and ethnic diversity. Focusing again on a number of specific countries, the chapters here highlight the challenges of crossing multiple boundaries between nation states, professional groups and the gendered division of labour in healthcare.

In Chapter Eleven Rannveig Dahle and Gry Skogheim consider the notion of flexibilisation and the implementation of the new public management, using agency nurses in Norway as an example, as well as potential gender traps in the nursing profession. Katalin Formadi in Chapter Twelve examines cross-mobility in the emerging field of employment in the health and wellness tourist sector in Hungary, thereby extending the notion of professional development to a sector currently outside the scope of public control. Joana Sousa Ribeiro in Chapter Thirteen, on the other hand, provides some interesting insights into foreign health professionals in Portugal from the viewpoint of migration and occupational integration. Finally, in Chapter Fourteen, Elianne Riska and Aurelija Novelskaite use survey and interview data to analyse the views of female and male physicians in Lithuania on intentions to migrate, and highlight the gendered mobility track of the health workforce.

In the Conclusion, the editors pull together the various threads of the collection by considering the future of health policy and workforce dynamics in rethinking professional governance in the international context. This is aimed at further enhancing the coherence of the book, which had its origin in a specially invited workshop on 'Professions, globalisation and the European project: shifting spheres of opportunity' held under the auspices of the European Sociological Association Sociology of Professions Research Network at the University of Bremen in April/May 2006. The volume mainly draws on selected contributions to this workshop, complemented by a small number of additional contributions. The editors wish sincerely to thank all of the contributors for helping to produce this innovative edited collection, which adds further essential dimensions to current international research on professional governance in the health field.

References

Allsop, J. and Saks, M. (eds) (2002) *Regulating the health professions*, London: Sage Publications.

Baggott, R., Allsop, J. and Jones, K. (2004) *Speaking for patients and carers: Health consumer groups and the policy process*, Basingstoke: Palgrave.

Barnes, M., Newman, J. and Sullivan, H. (2007) *Policy, participation and political renewal*, Bristol: The Policy Press.

Blank, R.H. and Burau, V. (2004) *Comparative health policy*, Houndmills: Palgrave.

Blank, R.H. and Burau, V. (2007) *Comparative health policy* (2nd edition), Houndmills: Palgrave.

Bourgeault, I.L. and Mulvale, G. (2006) 'Collaborative health care teams in Canada and the US: confronting the structural embeddedness of medical dominance', *Health Sociology Review*, vol 15, no 5, pp 481-95.

Burau, V. and Blank, R.H. (2006) 'Comparing health policy: an assessment of typologies of health systems', *Journal of Comparative Policy Analysis*, vol 8, pp 63-76.

Clarke, J. (2004) *Changing welfare, changing states: New directions in social policy*, London: Sage Publications.

Clarke, J., Newman, J., Smith, V., Vidler, E. and Westmarland, L. (2007) *Creating citizen-consumers: Changing publics, changing public services*, London: Sage Publications.

Davies, C. (2006) 'Heroes of health care? Replacing the medical profession in the policy process in the UK', in J.W. Duyvendak, T. Knijn and M. Kremer (eds) *Policy, people and the new professional*, Amsterdam: Amsterdam University Press, pp 137-51.

Davies, C., Wetherell, M. and Barnett, E. (2006) *Citizens at the centre: Deliberative participation in healthcare decisions*, Bristol: The Policy Press.

Dent, M. (2003) *Remodelling hospitals and health professions in Europe*, Houndmills: Palgrave.

DH (Department of Health) (2006) *Good doctors, safer patients*, London: The Stationery Office.

DH (2007) *Trust assurance and safety – the regulation of health professionals in the 21st century*, London: The Stationery Office.

Dubois, A., McKee, M. and Nolte, E. (eds) (2006) *Human resources for health in Europe*, Milton Keynes: Open University Press.

Duyvendak, J.W., Knijn, T. and Kremer, M. (eds) (2006) *Policy, people and the new professional: De-professionalisation and re-professionalisation in care and welfare*, Amsterdam: Amsterdam University Press.

Evetts, J. (2006) 'Introduction: trust and professionalism: challenges and occupational changes', *Current Sociology*, vol 54, no 4, pp 607-20.

Freidson, E. (2001) *Professionalism: The third logic*, Oxford: Polity Press.

Gray, A. and Harrison, S. (eds) (2004) *Governing medicine: Theory and practice*, Milton Keynes: Open University Press.

Hunter, D.J. (2006) 'From tribalism to corporatism: the continuing managerial challenge to medical dominance', in D. Kelleher, J. Gabe, and G. Williams (eds) *Challenging medicine* (2nd edition), London: Routledge, pp 1-23.

Hvinden, B. and Johansson, H. (eds) (2007) *Citizenship in Nordic welfare states: Dynamics of choice, duties and participation in a changing Europe*, London: Routledge.

Johnson, T., Larkin, G. and Saks, M. (eds) (1995) *Health professions and the state in Europe*, London: Routledge.

Kuhlmann, E. (2006) *Modernising health care: Reinventing professions, the state and the public*, Bristol: The Policy Press.

McDonald, R. and Harrison, S. (2004) 'The micropolitics of clinical guidelines: an empirical study', *Policy & Politics*, vol 13, pp 223-39.

Maynard, A. and Street, A. (2006) 'Seven years of feast, seven years of famine: boom to bust in the NHS?', *British Medical Journal*, vol 332, pp 906-8.

Moran, M. (1999) *Governing the health care state*, Manchester: Manchester University Press.

Mossialos, E. and McKee, M. (2002) 'Editorial: health care and the European Union. Profound uncertain consequences for national health systems', *British Medical Journal*, vol 324, pp 991-2.

Newman, J. (2005) 'Introduction', in J. Newman (ed) *Remaking governance: Peoples, politics and the public sphere*, Bristol: The Policy Press, pp 1-15.

Newman, J. and Kuhlmann, E. (2007) 'Consumers enter the political stage? Modernization of health care in Britain and Germany', *European Journal of Social Policy*, vol 17, no 2, pp 99-111.

Raak, A., Paulus, A. and Mur-Veeman, I. (2005) 'Why do health and social care providers cooperate?', *Health Policy*, vol 74, pp 13-23.

Riska, E. (2001) *Medical careers and feminist agendas: American, Scandinavian, and Russian women physicians*, New York: Aldine de Gruyter.

Room, G. (2007) 'Challenges facing the EU: scope for a coherent response', *European Societies*, vol 9, no 2, pp 229-44.

Saks, M. and Allsop, J. (eds) (2007) *Researching health: Qualitative, quantitative and mixed methods*, London: Sage Publications.

Saks, M. and Kuhlmann, E. (2006) 'Introduction. Professions, social inclusion and citizenship: challenge and change in European health systems', *Knowledge, Work and Society*, vol 4, no 1, pp 9-20.

Salter, B. (2002) 'Medical regulation: new politics and old power structures', *Politics*, vol 22, no 2, pp 59-67.

Sicotte, C., D'Amour, D. and Moreault, M.-P. (2002) 'Interdisciplinary collaboration within Quebec community health care centres', *Social Science and Medicine*, vol 55, pp 991-1003.

Vabø, M. (2006) 'Caring for people or caring for proxy consumers?', *European Societies*, vol 8, no 3, pp 403-22.

Waring, J. (2007) 'Adaptive regulation or governmentality: patient safety and the changing regulation of medicine', *Sociology of Health and Illness*, vol 29, no 2, pp 163-79.

Witz, A. and Annandale, E. (2006) 'The challenge of nursing', in D. Kelleher, J. Gabe and G. Williams (eds) *Challenging medicine* (2nd edition), London: Routledge, pp 24-39.

Wrede, S., Benoit, C., Bourgeault, I., van Teijlingen, E., Sandall, J. and De Vries, R. (2006) 'Decentred comparative research: context sensitive analysis of maternal health care', *Social Science and Medicine*, vol 63, pp 2986-97.

Xyrichis, A. and Lowton, K. (forthcoming) 'What fosters or prevents interprofessional teamwork in primary and community care? A literature review', *International Journal of Nursing Studies*, available online at doi:10.1016/j.ijnurstu.2007.01.015.

Part One
New directions in the governance of healthcare

ONE

Protecting patients: international trends in medical governance

Judith Allsop and Kathryn Jones

Introduction

The regulation of professional work in healthcare has become tighter as states aim to provide cost-effective, high-quality health services for citizens. This is particularly true in the case of medical professionals whose clinical decisions generate substantial healthcare spending. In consequence, a variety of institutions, rules and regulations have developed across countries that aim to control and shape the decision making of physicians. Although the aims are similar, the mechanisms differ as they are shaped by history and culture. The extent of professional self-government, the range of functions that come within the scope of self-governance and the institutional regulators vary between health systems. In this chapter the focus is on the role played by professional regulators in governing their own activities. The emphasis here is on the medical profession although reforms also affect other health professions. This is either because they are included in reforming legislation, or there is a trickle-down effect as other professions follow the medical model. A key question for policy makers has been how to hold the health professions accountable for achieving good-quality care. For professional regulators, key questions have been how to maintain the continuing competence of professionals throughout their careers and how to identify poor performance early in order to protect the public.

This chapter considers the trends in professional governance in order to identify the similarities and differences in addressing these key questions. It draws on a research study (Allsop and Jones, 2006a) that contributed to a wider review of professional governance in the UK following the final report of the Shipman Inquiry (2005) into how former general practitioner Harold Shipman was able to murder over 200 of his patients. The review undertaken by the Chief Medical Officer recommended radical changes in professional governance in the UK that are currently being implemented (DH, 2007). The research study looked at New South Wales, Australia; Ontario, Canada; Finland; France; the Netherlands; New Zealand; and New York State in the United States (US). These case studies were selected on two criteria: the countries had different forms of health system and were identified as being at the forefront of innovation in the literature. For non-English-speaking countries, experts were identified to contribute to our review.

The chapter briefly considers theories of self-regulation and background factors that have led to a challenge to professional governance prior to examining the similarities and differences in reform strategies. The conclusion comments on the implications of change for medical and, by extension, health professionals.

The theory and practice of self-regulation

As scholars of the professions have pointed out, due to the expert nature of medical work, and the status of healthcare as both a social service and a private good, regulatory authority has been vested in self-regulatory professional, as well as state, institutions. These vary between countries and, as Dubois and colleagues (2006) argue, there is a continuum in the extent of direct state control and the exercise of professional autonomy as well as variation in the areas in which state control or professional autonomy is exercised. In countries where professional self-regulation has been the norm, professional associations tend to set the rules to control who is certified to practise by keeping a register; determine what standards of practice there should be by issuing guidelines; and take disciplinary action where practitioners fall below those standards. Put another way, professional associations have tended to dominate knowledge creation through research, knowledge transmission through education and knowledge application through regulating standards (Salter, 1999). In countries where this is not the case, medical professionals work within state bureaucracies with varying degrees of autonomy to set policy.

Taking the countries within the review, in Australia, Canada, France and New Zealand key functions are carried out by an elected professional body. In Finland, the Netherlands and the US state bodies maintain registers of those qualified and discipline practitioners but professional associations play a major role in determining the standards for specialist care. Typically, regulation is nested in wider health systems funded through taxation and public and private insurance bringing a network of regulators that is more, or less, well articulated at the micro, meso and macro level. The role of insurers as a buffer between the state and the medical profession provides an interesting area of investigation, but is beyond the scope of this chapter.

The boundary between what should be under direct state control and what areas of practice should be determined by a self-regulating medical profession and the representation of interests has been contested in both theory and practice (Macdonald, 1995). Functionalist theorists and professional elites have argued for self-regulation on the grounds that the profession is in the best position to offset knowledge asymmetry and self-police standards and can do so at lower cost (see Abbott, 1988; Tallis, 2005). Critics have seen such claims as self-interested and have argued that monopoly powers tend to promote private interests rather than altruism and the public good (Freidson, 1970). Elected professional groups may be subject to regulatory capture by groups within their membership and the public interest may be displaced by group interests (Gellhorn, 1976; Stacey, 1992). In addition, empirical research has shown the particular difficulties in regulating medical practice. The course of disease varies in individuals and there are uncertainties in diagnosis, treatment and outcomes (Bosk, 1979).

The changing context of medical practice

Despite intermittent public criticism, traditional forms of professionally dominated regulation have been slow to change. Over the past decades, however, alongside policy makers' concerns to achieve cost-effective healthcare, various factors have combined to bring medical autonomy and self-regulation into question such as: the perception of medicine as a 'high-risk industry'; advances in evidence-based practice; the failures of regulators to detect poor practice; and the increasing complexity of the regulatory task in nation states. First, following research into the incidence of adverse events, hospital-based medicine in particular is ranked as a high-risk activity alongside aviation and nuclear power processing (DH, 2006; Flin, 2006). Based mainly on the examination of medical records, studies in the US (Brennan et al, 1991; Leape et al, 1991; Thomas et al, 2000), Australia (Wilson et al, 1995; Runciman et al, 2000), New Zealand (Davis et al, 2001) and the UK (Vincent et al, 2001) show the incidence of 'avoidable errors' to range from around 4% of hospital admissions (in the US) to 17% (in Australia). Methodological differences in the studies may account for some of the variation (Runciman et al, 2000).

Policy makers and regulators have responded to these data by seeking to increase providers' awareness of risk. For instance, the influential US report *To err is human* (Kohn et al, 1999) recommended targets for reducing error, and in a number of countries adverse incident reporting systems have been strengthened so that lessons may be learnt. For example, in the UK, the National Patient Safety Agency (NPSA) analyses reports from health and primary care trusts on adverse events. Similar agencies exist in other countries for accreditation and safety purposes. Professional associations, particularly the medical specialties, may also document adverse events (see DH, 2006). The change in perceptions and priorities is reflected in the language used by professionals and policy makers and, in our review, we found that most professional regulatory bodies now state that their aim is to protect patient safety (Allsop and Jones, 2006a, 2006b). How effective these systems are is another question.

A second and linked factor focusing on medical practice standards has been the development of evidence-based medicine. Some forms of intervention are 'more effective' than others, and therefore provide a preferred form of treatment. International agencies such as the Cochrane Collaboration promote information sharing. Across nation states, agencies have been established to assess current knowledge and produce guidelines on recommended diagnostic and therapeutic procedures such as the UK National Institute for Health and Clinical Excellence (NICE). Similar agencies exist in other countries to promote accreditation, safety and guideline development, such as the Haute Autorité de Santé (HAS) in France, the Agency for Healthcare Research and Quality in the US and the Australian Commission on Standards and Quality in Health Care. Both defences and critiques of evidence-based and target-driven bureaucratic-scientific medicine have been mounted (Timmermans and Berg, 2003; Beenamouzig and Besançon, 2005; Goldenberg, 2006; Lambert et al, 2006). For the purposes of the argument here, some therapies have been well validated and the wide variations in practice that were part and parcel of clinical autonomy are no longer tolerated. The implication for physicians is that they must update their knowledge to keep abreast of current practice. Our review found that the case for continued updating was accepted across the countries in our study as well as in the UK. This agenda has been pursued in different ways and strategies are discussed further below.

In some countries, a third factor bringing medical competence and professional governance onto the policy agenda has been individual instances of seriously poor performance, often of a serial nature, that have harmed patients. The inquiries and publicity associated with these cases have placed a spotlight on previously opaque decision making within self-regulatory bodies. In the UK, the inquiry into children's heart surgery at the Bristol Royal Infirmary (Bristol Inquiry, 2001), the Shipman Inquiry (2005) and others (see DH, 2006, p viii); in Australia, the inquiry into long-stay care homes in New South Wales (1990) and the ongoing inquiry into deaths at Queensland's Bundaberg Hospital (Van der Weyden, 2005); and, in New Zealand, the inquiry into poorly designed research on cervical cancer (Cartwright Inquiry, 1998) have led to seismic changes in medical regulation. They have served to strengthen existing concerns about the efficacy of self-regulation leading to calls for greater transparency and accountability.

A final factor leading to change has been the recognition among professional regulators themselves that the complexity of the regulatory task itself has increased and that membership institutions – many of which were established in the 19th century – may no longer be fit for purpose. Public expectations and standards have risen so that professional regulators have had to develop and update their standards and guidelines for practice. Technological advances in medicine have required new guidance on a range of ethical issues; the increasing mobility of medical graduates has expanded the administrative task of checking on qualifications, running examinations and ensuring that a person struck off the register does not then move to practise in another jurisdiction. The emergence of supranational governance organisations, such as the World Federation of Medical Education and the European Accreditation Council for Continuing Medical Education, has also widened the scope of regulatory activity. In the course of responding to the regulatory challenge, at least in the UK, the professional governance body has tended to become remote from rank-and-file physicians and open to criticism from its own professional elites (Smith, 1992; Irvine, 2003).

Trends in professional governance

Across countries, several trends in professional governance can be identified. Since the 1990s, many states have introduced legislation to modernise arrangements, typically justifying change in terms of protecting patients and assuring high-quality healthcare. It is also common for legislation to include a range of health professions as well as medicine within a common legislative framework, thus giving parity, at least symbolically, to all the health professions, rather than setting medicine apart (see also Boyce, this volume).

In Ontario in Canada the 1991 Regulated Health Professions Act related to 20 professions; in the Netherlands the 1996 Individual Health Care Professions Act (BIG Act) covered eight professions and brought changes to disciplinary procedures; and in New Zealand 15 professions are regulated under the 2003 Health Practitioners' Competence Act. In Australia (New South Wales) the 1992 Medical Practice Act reconfigured physician regulation and in 1993 the Health Care Complaints Act provided a common framework for the pursuit of complaints against different health professions. In Finland the health and welfare professions that provide public services were already regulated within a government department. In the UK there is currently a lack of uniformity between the health professions as their statutes of self-governance reflect past conventions. The 2002 Health Act established the Council for Healthcare Regulatory Excellence, which is charged with increasing the consistency of regulation across the health professions. One of these, the Health Professions Council, itself regulates 13 professions within a common framework (Walshe and Benson, 2005; Allsop and Jones, 2006b). It is worth noting that only two of the countries in our study – Canada and the Netherlands – license particular professionals to carry out specific, named tasks. In other countries, regulatory bodies register professionals on the basis of their qualification to use a specific title that implicitly confers an ability to carry out certain procedures.

Where countries have passed recent legislation, this has sometimes included changes in the composition of the governing body to replace elected members entirely with appointments by government, as in New South Wales in Australia and New Zealand. Currently, professional governing bodies in Canada, the UK and France are mainly elected membership bodies. For the UK the Donaldson review (DH, 2006) has recommended an appointed council to replace the current General Medical Council (GMC). Arrangements in the US have always varied widely and in New York State the state medical board has long been an appointed body. In most countries, governing councils have included lay appointees whose numbers over time have tended to increase as a proportion of the membership. There has also been a trend towards increasing the accountability of professional governing councils to the legislature. This is currently the case in Finland, Canada, New South Wales in Australia and New Zealand and is to be adopted in the UK (DH, 2007).

Assessing professional competence

Another trend in medical regulation has been the establishment of codes of conduct and professional standards that set out what is expected of doctors. In the past, this has taken the form of general aspirational guidelines such as the GMC's recently updated *Good medical practice* (GMC, 2006), which outlines current best practice. However, in a number of countries policy makers have been working towards some form of periodic reassessment of physicians during their career to ensure that their knowledge and skills continue to meet an acceptable standard and healthcare quality is assured (Klazinga, 2000). Currently, the terminology for this process is not stable across English-speaking countries and translation adds further difficulties. Re-licensing or re-registration tends to be used when referring to the renewal of a physician's licence to practise. It may be annual and does not require any form of structured review or assessment. Re-accreditation usually refers to re-accrediting a physician as a member of their specialty association or college. Revalidation has been used in the UK to refer to a formal process for revalidating periodically a doctor's registration with the GMC. However, the terms can be used interchangeably. It is worth noting that a recent survey of public perceptions of medical regulation in the UK (MORI, 2005) found that a majority of members of the public believed that doctors' continuing competence was already regularly reviewed by the GMC. This is not the case, and became politically contentious when the Shipman Inquiry (2005) criticised heavily the GMC's then current proposals for revalidation.

Two approaches to maintaining physicians' competence have developed: the learning model and the assessment model. Our cross-country review found that continuing medical education (CME) or continuing professional development (CPD) as a learning model has become policy across all the countries reviewed. However, programmes vary in terms of who decides the content and appropriateness of courses; who takes responsibility for providing them; whether they are compulsory; the sanctions for non-compliance; and how learning outcomes are monitored.

In countries where physicians must re-license with their regulatory body annually, a statement on participation in CME/CPD as well as any complaints or claims may be required. In others, employers and/or health insurers may require evidence of CME. Typically, the professional specialty associations have played a major role in developing and monitoring programmes and there may be requirements for continuing membership. University medical schools may also be providers (as in the Netherlands) or central government (as in the French regions, initiated by the Haute Autorité de Santé – see Allsop and Jones, 2006a). However, participation in CME may be tokenistic, 'gaming' may be widespread (Bevan and Hood, 2005) and there is insufficient evidence that participation maintains competence.

Due to the drawbacks of the learning model, a number of countries are moving towards periodic review and assessment of physicians' competence, usually every five to ten years. Currently, the two main approaches to assessment are either through a computer-based multi-module programme or through face-to-face peer review using standardised instruments. Both approaches are professionally led and aim to assess a range of skills, knowledge and competencies covering, for example, clinical diagnostic skills, communicating with patients and relatives, teamwork and practice management, and both work with the concept of a threshold of competence to be reached.

The first of these approaches has been most fully developed in the US, where around 85% of physicians practise as specialists. Specialist accreditation is required by health insurers and employers and there are financial incentives to encourage physicians to seek re-accreditation where their specialty has developed programmes. Currently, the nationwide specialty boards are at different stages of development although the American Board of Medical Specialties has set out a common framework for 'Maintenance of Certification' programmes. This sets out six competencies across four components – professional standing, professional performance, lifelong learning through self-assessment and cognitive expertise – assessed over a 10-year cycle.

In 1991, the Netherlands launched a mandatory, peer-led scheme for specialist re-registration to maintain quality. Run by a coordinating body, the College of Specialists, it now covers 27 specialties including general practice and, since 2005, has been based on three criteria for re-registration: physicians must practise their specialty for a minimum number of hours per week; they must take part in CME to gain accreditation points; and every five years they must participate in a peer-led 'visitatie' programme that reviews individual and team practice (Lombarts and Van Wijmen, 2003). Instruments have been developed for a multidimensional evaluation covering standards of clinical care; an assessment of specialty professional development; and an assessment from the patient perspective. The aim is to make the process objective, but professionally led. In France, the Haute Autorité de Santé has launched a broadly similar specialty-led accreditation system centrally for the hospital sector that includes periodic physician evaluation. This now covers independent specialists and generalists (les medécins liberaux). For generalists, the scheme is to be led by the regional professional association, and allows the physician discretion to choose their reviewer. It is in a very early stage of development. For the UK, the locally based system recommended for 're-accrediting' physicians is likely to take the form of a 360-degree review, involving peers, the public and managers (DH, 2006).

Identifying and acting on poor performance

Health regulators across countries are also concerned with the problem of identifying physicians whose work falls below an acceptable standard. This may mean removing them from practice to protect patients. Until recently, in all but two of the countries in our review, disciplinary matters were investigated and dealt with by the professional body. The exceptions are the US, where professionally dominated state boards undertake this function and in Finland, where responsibility lies with a government department. When sanctions were applied, these were severe, but applied relatively rarely. Research on fitness to practise procedures has been limited, procedures opaque and comparative studies virtually non-existent (Ameringer, 1999; Salter, 1999; Allsop, 2002); however, certain trends are discernible.

Most countries have introduced procedures to deal with physicians whose performance is impaired through ill-health, and, typically, this has been a function of the professional body with responsibility for registration. The approach has been rehabilitative. Physicians are encouraged to step down from practice voluntarily, receive treatment and support, returning to practise when they are fit. More recently, this approach has been extended to physicians whose performance comes to the attention of the regulatory body and is assessed as falling below an acceptable standard. Physicians who do not comply with informal processes are dealt with through the disciplinary process.

The strategies used by the professional regulatory body to identify poor performance vary between countries. In Canada, the provinces have adopted an approach that combines routine performance assessments for accreditation for all physicians with, if problems are identified, subsequent in-depth assessments. Currently, there is variation in the detail between provinces. For example, Alberta has a rolling programme of practice assessments with two levels of further assessment for practitioners found to be performing poorly. In Ontario, 10% of all practices are assessed annually, and practitioners over the age of 70 every five years. In Quebec, physicians are selected for review if they are identified as statistical outliers on a range of indicators (for example, in prescribing patterns, immunisation records and the identification of chronic illness). A characteristic of these schemes is that they are profession led and rehabilitation programmes are organised by professional bodies in collaboration with the regulatory body.

As far as public protection is concerned, one of the disadvantages of professional bodies dealing with poor performance is that they tend to be unaccountable and lack transparency on the standards used to identify poor practice and the criteria and thresholds used for referral. For example, the final report of the Shipman Inquiry (2005) contained sharp criticism of the GMC, by the Chair, Dame Janet Smith, a High Court judge, for the lack of clear processes in the fitness to practise procedures.

State agencies as well as public and private health insurers also have an interest in identifying poor practice. For example, in the US, claims, complaints and poor treatment outcomes can lead to physicians losing their accreditation status. In public insurance-based systems, agencies may scrutinise reimbursement claims to identify physicians whose performance is significantly out of line with practice norms, or is fraudulent. Cases may be referred on to the regulatory body. New agencies have also been established in some countries to provide an assessment service for employers supplementing and complementing the role of the professional regulatory body, such as the UK NPSA and, in the US, the Institute for Physician Evaluation. It is estimated in the UK that between 0.5% of all doctors and 1% of senior doctors are referred to the NPSA annually. About 10% of these go through a complete assessment (DH, 2006).

In New Zealand and New South Wales in Australia the close informal cooperation between the Medical Council and the Health and Disciplinary Commissioner who deals with complaints helps to ensure joint decisions on which institution should deal with a case. The investigations undertaken by the Health and Disciplinary Commissioner are particularly thorough. Reports are publicly available and any lessons learnt from an investigation that can be applied to medical practice in general are widely disseminated (Allsop and Jones, 2006a).

These developments signal, in the terminology of Foucault (see Dean, 1999), the widening scope of the 'disciplinary gaze'. They also indicate extensive network governance systems justified in terms of public protection (Clarke and Newman, 1997). This is apparent too in relation to physicians against whom some sort of legal or disciplinary action has been taken. The US federal government maintains a National Surveillance Data Bank that can be used by employers and other officials to check credentials and there are also other commercial data banks that can be accessed by consumers. The reliability of these information sources depends on the accuracy of reporting. Indeed, Holtman (2007) argues that the system of medical licensure in the US is fragmentary with little oversight by the federal government, because licensure and disciplinary action are determined at state level.

At the international level, there is now collaboration in information exchange between health regulators as a consequence of concerns about errant physicians struck off the register in one country moving to practise in another, through such organisations as the International Association of Medical Regulatory Authorities (IAMRA). Health regulators remain concerned about possible loopholes in existing arrangements as physician migration and bilateral and multilateral agreements encouraging the free movement of labour increase. The Alliance of Health Regulators in Europe (AURE) brings together 10 health and social care regulators in the UK to work together on issues affecting patient and client safety.

The different ways of dealing with poor performance are linked to national institutional structures and professional politics that are often resistant to change (see Cuperus-Bosma et al, 2006). However, our cross-country review showed that in a number of countries the final stage of the disciplinary process where a physician may be removed from practice has been transferred from the professional regulatory body to an independent tribunal, often covering other health professionals and chaired by a lawyer, with panel members of professionals and the laity. New Zealand, New South Wales in Australia and the US at state level follow this model, and the Donaldson review (DH, 2006) has recommended a similar model for the medical profession in the UK.

Conclusion

Our review of medical regulation has shown that reforms are taking place across countries that are broadly similar in response to the drive towards higher-quality, safer healthcare. Although the strategies are different, periodic assessment of competence during a physician's career and the early identification of poor performance are developing across countries, albeit at different stages of evolution. In many countries, new agencies have developed so that partnership or network regulation for all the health professions as well as medicine is common. Some institutions are state led, others are run by the profession, but partnership or network governance "within and between nation states is becoming the norm" (see Burau and Vrangbæk, this volume). "This requires cooperation between professionals and between professionals and other regulators." Formal accountability of the professional body to elected governments is also more extensive and direct. In most countries, disciplinary action that may result in a physician being removed from practice now tends to be the responsibility of a specialist tribunal.

One conclusion from our review of medical regulation in different countries is that the profession is no longer a judge in its own case. How these new institutional forms operate in practice, to what kind of standards and with what outcome, remains to be explored. A second important conclusion: to date, change appears to have been achieved without overt conflict between governments and the medical profession. This may be because the task of professional governance has moved beyond the capacity of the traditional professional membership body or because rank-and-file professionals have become distanced from their regulatory body. It may also be that physicians identify mainly with their specialty association.

Furthermore, in tax-based systems, healthcare is already heavily regulated; and surveillance has increased in publicly and privately based insurance systems. In most countries, medical professionals have maintained both status and income. Nevertheless, difficulties remain in identifying physicians who are performing poorly. Methods differ widely across countries. There are cultural barriers to colleague reporting. Managers may be unable to judge clinical practice or lack the power to intervene. Some doctors are in solo practice and to date little research has been undertaken into factors that can act as early warning signs of later poor performance.

In sum, in many countries, professional elites have taken responsibility for and control of physician assessment for periodic re-certification or re-accreditation. The tools used for assessment and the conduct of reviews remain in the hands of professionals. However, the notion that standards of practice across a number of domains can be identified and assessed either objectively by testing, or more subjectively through peer review, has had profound repercussions for the practice of medicine as well as for other health professions and their regulators. How the different methods play out between specialties and across countries should be fertile ground for future researchers.

References

Abbott, A. (1988) *The system of professions: An essay on the division of expert labor*, Chicago, IL: University of Chicago Press.

Allsop, J. (2002) 'Regulating the medical profession', in J. Allsop and M. Saks (eds) *Regulating the health professions*, London: Sage Publications, pp 79-93.

Allsop, J. and Jones, K. (2006a) *Quality assurance in medical regulation in an international context*, Lincoln: University of Lincoln.

Allsop, J. and Jones, K. (2006b) 'The regulation of the health care professions: towards greater partnership between the state, professions and citizens in the UK', *Knowledge, Work and Society*, vol 4, no 1, pp 35-58.

Ameringer, C.F. (1999) *State medical boards and the politics of public protection*, Baltimore, MA: Johns Hopkins University Press.

Beenamouzig, D. and Besançon, J. (2005) 'Administrer un monde incertain: les nouvelles bureaucraties techniques: le cas des agences sanitaires en France', *Sociologie du Travail*, vol 47, no 3, pp 301-22.

Bevan, G. and Hood, C. (2005) *What is measured is what matters: Targets and gaming in the English public health care system*, ESRC Public Services Programme, Discussion Paper Series no. 0501, http://public-services.politics.ox.ac.uk/Publications/Bevan_v2.pdf

Bosk, C. (1979) *Forgive and remember: Managing medical failure*, Chicago, IL: University of Chicago Press.

Brennan, T.A., Leape, L.L., Laird, N.M., Hebert, L., Localio, A.R., Lawthers, A.G., Newhouse, J.P., Weiler, P.C. and Hiatt, H.H. (1991) 'Incidence of adverse events and negligence in hospitalised patients: the results of the Harvard Medical Practice Study I', *New England Journal of Medicine*, vol 324, pp 370-6.

Bristol Inquiry (2001) *Learning from Bristol, Public Inquiry into Children's Heart Surgery at the Bristol Royal Infirmary 1984-1995*, London: The Stationery Office.

Cartwright Inquiry, Dame Silvia (1998) *The Report of the Committee of Inquiry into Allegations Concerning the Treatment of Cervical Cancer at National Women's Hospital*, Auckland: WHA.

Clarke, J. and Newman, J. (1997) *The managerial state*, London: Sage Publications.

Cuperus-Bosma, J., Hout, F., Hubben, J. and van der Val, G. (2006) 'The views of physicians, disciplinary board members and practising lawyers on the new statutory disciplinary system for health care in the Netherlands', *Health Policy*, vol 77, pp 202-11.

Davis, P., Lay-Yee, R., Briant, R., Ali, W., Scott, A. and Schug, S. (2001) 'Adverse events regional feasibility study: indicative findings', *New Zealand Medical Journal*, vol 114, pp 203-5.

Dean, M. (1999) *Governmentality: Power and rule in modern society*, London: Sage Publications.

DH (Department of Health) (2006) *Good doctors, safer patients: Proposals to strengthen the system to assure and improve the performance of doctors and to protect the safety of patients*, London: The Stationery Office.

DH (Department of Health) (2007) *Trust assurance and safety: The regulation of health professionals*, London: The Stationery Office.

Dubois, C.-A., Dixon, A. and McKee, M. (2006) 'Reshaping the regulation of the workforce in European health care systems', in C.-A. Dubois, M. McKee and E. Nolte (eds) *Human resources for health in* Europe, Milton Keynes: Open University Press, pp 173-92.

Flin, R. (2006) *Safe in their hands: Licensing and quality assessment for safety-critical roles in high risk industries*, Aberdeen: University of Aberdeen, www.abdn.ac.uk/iprc/papers%20reports/Safe_In_Their_Hands_Revalidation_Report.pdf

Freidson, E. (1970) *Profession of medicine: A study of the sociology of applied knowledge*, New York: Dodd, Mead & Co.

Gellhorn, W. (1976) 'The abuse of occupational licensing', *University of Chicago Law Review*, vol 44, pp 6-27.

GMC (General Medical Council) (2006) *Good medical practice*, London: GMC, www.gmc-uk.org/guidance/good_medical_practice/GMC_GMP_V41.pdf

Goldenberg, M. (2006) 'On evidence and evidence-based medicine: lessons from the philosophy of science', *Social Science and Medicine*, vol 62, pp 2621-32.

Holtman, M.C. (2007) 'Disciplinary careers of drug-impaired physicians', *Social Science and Medicine*, vol 64, pp 509-20.

Irvine, D. (2003) *The doctors' tale: Professionalism and public trust*, Abingdon: Radcliffe Medical Press.

Klazinga, N. (2000) 'Re-engineering trust: the adoption and adaptation of four models for external quality assurance of health care services in Western European health care systems', *International Journal for Quality in Health Care*, vol 13, no 3, pp 183-9.

Kohn, L.T., Corrigan, J.M. and Donaldson, M.S. (eds) (1999) *To err is human: Building a safer healthcare system*, Washington, DC: Institute of Medicine, National Academy Press.

Lambert, H., Gordon, E.J. and Bogdan-Lovis, E.A. (2006) 'Introduction: Gift horse or Trojan horse? Social science perspectives on evidence-based health care', *Social Science and Medicine*, vol 62, pp 2613-20.

Leape, L.L., Brennan, T.A., Laird, N.M., Lawthers, A.G., Localio, A.R., Barnes, B.A., Hebert, L., Newhouse, J.P., Weiler, P.C. and Hiatt, H.H. (1991) 'The nature of adverse events in hospitalized patients: results of the Harvard Medical Practice Study II', *New England Journal of Medicine*, vol 324, pp 377-94.

Lombarts, M.J. and Van Wijmen, F.C. (2003) 'External peer review by medical specialist (visitatie) in a legal perspective', *European Journal of Health Law*, vol 10, no 1, pp 43-51.

Macdonald, K. (1995) *The sociology of the professions*, London: Sage Publications.

MORI (2005) *Attitudes to medical regulation and revalidation of doctors*, London: MORI, www.mori.com/polls/2005/pdf/doh.pdf

New South Wales (1990) *Report of the Royal Commission into Deep Sleep Therapy: The Honourable Acting Justice J.P. Slattery*, Sydney: The Commission.

Runciman, W.B., Webb, R.K., Helps, S.C., Thomas, E.J., Sexton, E.S., Studdert, D.M. and Brennan, T.A. (2000) 'A comparison of iatrogenic injury studies in Australia and the USA reviewer behaviour and quality of care', *International Journal of Quality in Health Care*, vol 12, no 5, pp 379-88.

Salter, B. (1999) *Medical regulation and public trust: An international review*, London, King's Fund Publishing.

Shipman Inquiry (2005) *Safeguarding patients: Lessons from the past – proposals for the future. Fifth Report*, Manchester: The Shipman Inquiry, www.the-shipman-inquiry.org.uk/fifthreport.asp

Smith, R. (1992) 'The GMC on performance: professional self-regulation is on the line', *British Medical Journal*, vol 304, p 1257.

Stacey, M. (1992) *Regulating British medicine: The General Medical Council*, Chichester: Wiley.

Tallis, R. (2005) *Hippocratic oaths; medicine and its discontents*, London: Atlantic Books.

Thomas, E.J., Studdert, D.M., Burstin, H.R., Orav, E.J., Zeena, T., Williams, E.J., Howard, K.M., Weiler, P.C. and Brennan, T.A. (2000) 'Incidence and types of adverse events and negligence care in Utah and Colorado', *Medical Care*, vol 38, pp 261-71.

Timmermans, S. and Berg, M. (2003) *The gold standard: The challenge of evidence-based medicine and standardization in heath care*, Philadelphia, PA: Temple University Press.

Van der Weyden, M.B. (2005) 'The Bundaberg Hospital scandal: the need for reform in Queensland and beyond', *Medical Journal of Australia*, vol 183, no 6, pp 284-5.

Vincent, C., Neale, G. and Woloshynowych, M. (2001) 'Adverse events in British hospital: a preliminary retrospective review', *British Medical Journal*, vol 322, pp 1154-7.

Walshe, K. and Benson, L. (2005) 'Time for radical reform', *British Medical Journal*, vol 330, pp 1504-6.

Wilson, R.M., Runciman, W.B., Gibberd, R.W., Harrison, B.T., Newby, L. and Hamilton, J.D. (1995) 'The quality in Australian health care study', *Medical Journal of Australia*, vol 163, pp 458-71.

TWO

Global markets and national pathways of medical re-regulation[1]

Viola Burau and Karsten Vrangbæk

Introduction

The market enjoys global currency. In healthcare, the market has been central to reforms across many countries, as is evident from the prominence of managed competition. At the same time, experiences with markets in healthcare suggest that the reforms not only have included considerable re-regulation, but also that such re-regulation remains firmly embedded in country-specific contexts. The present chapter aims to open the black box of 'global markets' by identifying country-specific pathways of re-regulation in relation to markets in healthcare in a cross-country comparative perspective. The chapter does so by analysing sector-specific institutional contexts from a cross-country comparative perspective based on five countries – Britain, Denmark, Germany, Italy and Norway. Medical governance is closely related to redistributive policies, where the influence of country-specific institutions tends to be pertinent. At the same time, medical governance is subject to considerable policy pressures centring on tensions between public accountability and professional autonomy. Medical governance therefore provides a good basis for studying both the dynamics of governance and the difference institutions make.

We introduce an analytical distinction between three forms of governance: hierarchy, network-based governance and professional self-regulation. *Hierarchy* is based on formal authority and is concerned with control, standardisation and accountability. Centralised systems of standard setting and auditing are an example of this form of governance. *Network-based governance* is characterised by interdependent flows of power and focuses on adaptation and flexibility. An example of this form of governance is the negotiation of quality standards among purchaser, provider and professional organisations. In contrast, the market focuses on maximising output, and governing occurs through competition among multiple and more or less autonomous agencies. In principle, this makes for a more devolved policy process. Yet in practice, it is often the government that sets the goals and targets that form the basis for monitoring, inspecting and auditing the performance of sub-central agencies. Finally, *professional self-regulation* relies on expert authority and aims for professional control over practice. Clinical guidelines set by professional bodies are an example of this form of governance.

The analysis suggests two things. First, developments in all countries included in the study point to the fact that the new medical governance is indeed characterised by strong elements of hierarchy-based forms of governance, but ones that are combined with other modes of governing, often in the form of hybrids. This means that old and new forms of governing exist side by side and even strongly interact with each other. Second, although the developments in the five countries share some commonalities, there are important differences relating to the relative balance between forms of governance, the specific meaning of individual forms of governing together with the specific interaction between different forms of governance. These variations point to the importance of sector-specific type of institutions (the healthcare state, the relative decentralisation of governing arrangements and the normative institutions of medical authority) and the country-specific combinations in which they occur.

The analysis begins by critically reviewing different approaches to conceptualising the institutional contexts of medical governance. Against this background, the analysis then presents a comparison of the dynamics of medical governance in five selected European countries and identifies institutionally embedded pathways of change. The analysis concludes by critically reviewing the potentials and limitations of institutions for understanding the dynamics of contemporary governance.

Conceptualising the institutional context of medical governance

In terms of the contexts of the governance of doctors, sector-specific institutions related to healthcare are particularly important, although these are embedded in wider institutional contexts. The comparative literature often conceptualises such institutions by using the typology of healthcare systems. The typology is based on different forms of funding and the underlying assumption is that the funding of healthcare also has implications for the provision of healthcare (Nolte et al, 2005).

In the context of analysing medical governance and how it is changing, this typology is problematic. The typology is primarily concerned with how such health systems operate. In contrast, questions as to the power struggles underpinning the organisation of healthcare and the implications for the distribution and application of power remain unanswered. However, it is precisely these questions that are central to the study of governance. Further, the typology focuses on the funding of healthcare and as such excludes other key aspects of the organisation of healthcare. In relation to the governance of doctors, including provision is central, as this is the main interface between doctors and the organisation of healthcare.

Michael Moran (1999, 2000) tries to address these shortcomings by developing a typology of 'healthcare states'. The typology is explicitly concerned with the governance of healthcare. It distinguishes between consumption, provision and technology as the central areas of governing and presents the corresponding institutions of governing. The first two are particularly relevant in the context of the present analysis. The institutions related to the consumption of healthcare are concerned with the mechanisms that decide on the total volume of resources allocated to the financing of healthcare, and the mechanisms by which individual patients have access to services. In contrast, the institutions related to the provision of healthcare are related to the mechanisms for governing hospital care and doctors (especially different forms of private interest government). This reflects the centrality of hospitals and doctors for the politics of healthcare provision.

The concept of the healthcare state allows us to capture the organisation of healthcare in terms of the institutions of governance. Nevertheless, in the context of the present analysis, a number of limitations remain. First, the concept of the healthcare state captures the regulative element of institutions. The focus is on the relationship with other institutions of health governance and the extent to which hierarchy-based forms of governing circumscribe private interest government. However, considering the many normative aspects associated with governing medical performance (for example as reflected in the importance of informal professional networks), the institutions of private interest government need to be further unpacked. The normative elements of institutions are about norms and values; that is, conceptions about desirable goals and legitimate means to achieve these goals. Normative institutions form the conceptual images that create roles and standardised patterns for interaction (March and Olsen, 1989). Perceptions of professional authority are central here and formal education and professional networks help to define and sustain such norms and values. This also provides a stepping stone for linking institutions to actors as suggested by the notion of actor–centred governance (Burau, 2005).

Second, the concept of the healthcare state stresses the embeddedness of the institutions of healthcare in the institutions of the state, yet the state seems to emerge as a unitary organisational entity. However, in relation to healthcare in many countries, states are characterised by a considerable degree of decentralisation. This reflects the features of the broader polity states that are embedded in and/or recent reforms that have decentralised different aspects of health governance. Further, moving away from professional self-regulation and towards strengthening public accountability requires a certain concentration of power in governing arrangements (see more generally Newman, 2001). Here, the relative centralisation or decentralisation of the state in relation to healthcare is an important factor facilitating or constraining such developments.

The analysis

Having defined the institutional context the next question is how to study the impact that such institutions have on changes in medical governance. At a basic level this requires answering the following two questions: What are the pathways of governance that the respective institutional contexts lay out? To what extent do the recent changes in governing arrangements follow these pathways?

In understanding medical governance, medical performance is central for two main reasons. First, as doctors as professionals are about applying knowledge, performance is a key area governing medical work. Second, compared to education and research, performance is the area of governing doctors that has the most direct effect on the public (see also Allsop and Jones, this volume). This politicises the governance of performance and therefore makes performance an ideal focus for studying changes in medical governance.

The governance of medical performance is about setting and monitoring standards about medical treatment and diagnosis. The analysis distinguishes between broad ideal types of governing mechanisms in order to capture the dynamics of change: hierarchy, market, network and professional self-regulation. Here it is important not to treat the ideal types as static and/or exclusive, but instead to look for: changes within individual governing mechanisms (such as professional self-regulation, which includes stronger control of individual doctors); the changing balance of power between different (co-existing) types of governing mechanisms (such as the increasing importance of market-based governance in healthcare); and the existence of hybrid-governing mechanisms (such as professional autonomy the boundaries of which are circumscribed by hierarchy).

Institutional contexts of governing medical performance

The present section compares and contrasts the institutional contexts of governing medical performance (see Table 2.1). This provides the basis for outlining the respective pathways of governing medical performance in the next section.

In Britain as an entrenched command-and-control healthcare state, the (central) state dominates the governance of provision and consumption through controlling both the raising of funds from general taxation and the allocation of funds through a public management hierarchy. State power is also relatively centralised. Taken together this circumscribes the private interest government of doctors to a considerable extent and it exists as a parallel governing regime. In terms of the governance of medical performance more specifically, the public nature of hospital and primary care trusts offers a springboard for governing through performance management. As larger organisations, hospitals have traditionally been more susceptible to government influence. This is changing, however, with the inclusion of general practitioner (GP) practices into primary care trusts as larger organisational units. Strong hierarchy together with some elements of the market are the key here. The relative unconnectedness of the private interest government of doctors makes for strong professional self-regulation, but at the same time also provides leverage for the reform of professional self-regulation.

Table 2.1: Institutional contexts of the governance of medical performance

	Healthcare state	(De)centralisation	Normative institutions
Britain	Entrenched command and control	Centralised	Medical authority based on professional self-regulation
Italy	Insecure command and control	Decentralised	Medical authority based on private practice
Denmark	Entrenched command and control	Decentralised	Publicly embedded medical authority
Norway	Entrenched command and control	Centralised	Publicly embedded medical authority
Germany	Corporatist	Decentralised	Institutionalised medical authority

In relation to the first aspect, medical societies in particular emerge as strong private interest organisations with wide scope for professional self-regulation. In Britain, the 13 medical Royal Colleges and Faculties and their associated specialist societies play a significant role not only in the field of postgraduate education for which they have a formal responsibility, but also in setting the standards to be used in the implementation of any clinical governance policy (Salter, 2001). As the revalidation policy has developed, so the Royal Colleges have played a significant role with varying degrees of acceptance of the leadership of the General Medical Council (GMC) (Irvine, 2003; Salter, 2004). In sum, this means that the normative institutions associated with the private interest government of doctors can best be characterised as medical authority first and foremost, based on professional self-regulation.

The institutional set-up of the healthcare state in Italy in many ways resembles that in Britain, although the regional governments rather than the central government are central to the governance of consumption and provision, enjoying considerable autonomy (Tousijn, 2005). The 'public' nature of the management chain also provides important leverage for change, although it is often characterised by low efficiency. Crucially, however, the importance of private payments and private practice undermines the formal roles of regional government and Italy can be characterised as an insecure command-and-control healthcare state. Further, the private interest government of doctors appears to be complementary rather than parallel, not least as elements of professional self-regulation are part of the public management regime. The normative institutions associated with private interest government can be characterised as medical authority based on private practice, and this in part reflects the weakness of managerial culture and the importance of political parties. In terms of the governance of medical performance, this gives primacy to professional self-regulation and hierarchy-based forms of governing, although with the limits that the private element in healthcare puts on hierarchy, informal negotiations are likely to play a key intermediary role. This also provides doctors with numerous important points of access to influence.

Regional government is also central to the healthcare state in Denmark, notably in the form of democratically elected counties that are responsible for the funding and provision of healthcare. In contrast to Italy, the relations between regional and the central level are embedded in a strong and well-established system of decentralisation based on (formal) negotiations and consensus seeking. Nevertheless, in recent years funding has become an increasingly important means to exert pressure from the centre (Vrangbæk and Martinsen, 2005). As in Britain, Denmark can therefore also be characterised as an entrenched command-and-control healthcare state. In contrast to Britain, the statutory body of professional regulation is integrated into public management structures and this makes for highly constrained private interest government. The corresponding normative institutions are therefore best characterised as 'publicly embedded medical authority' whereby doctors are closely involved in negotiations and consensus finding, also leading to a high degree of compliance in implementation. The governance of medical performance therefore presents itself as a closely intertwined mix between (central/regional) hierarchy and negotiations. As in Italy, the negotiations also allow doctors to exert considerable influence that in part counterbalances the weakness of professional self-regulation. In contrast to Italy the negotiations in Denmark are more strongly institutionally integrated and there is a constant interplay between bottom-up and top-down initiatives (Pedersen, 2005; Vrangbæk and Martinsen, 2005).

The situation is similar in Norway, although the healthcare state is more centralised: central government is responsible for raising funding from taxation, for allocating funds through a public management hierarchy and for governing hospitals through appointed regional agencies. Governing arrangements are more decentralised in relation to primary care, which is the responsibility of the municipalities (Grytten et al, 2003). The distinction between the local and the national level thus continues to be central with respect to primary care. The Norwegian Doctors' Association also remains influential at the central level in relation to both sectors of provision. There is also a tradition for the medical society to work with the state rather than against it (Byrkjeflot and Neby, 2004), both formally through the association and more informally through the high professional status of medicine. This means that the main normative institution of doctors' private interest government is closely intertwined with public institutions in many areas, for instance through education, the licensing of specialists, and managerial and professional positions in central health administration, as well as through negotiating health policy.

In all the countries discussed so far, although to different extents, the state has a highly influential role in the governance of consumption and provision. This contrasts with Germany, where the (federal) state only has a regulatory role and where statutory organisations of insurance funds and doctors are instead dominant (for an overview see Busse and Riesberg, 2004; Rosenbrock and Gerlinger, 2004). Overall, Germany can be characterised as a corporatist healthcare state. Similarly to Denmark, formal negotiations (at federal and state level) are a central feature of the healthcare state, but crucially these explicitly involve doctors. This reflects the fact that private interest government extends beyond professional regulation and includes the allocation of funding. Private interest government is therefore more extensive, but this comes with a closer integration in healthcare governance and corresponding constraints. In terms of the associated normative institutions, this makes for highly institutionalised medical authority, also characterised by strong elements of private practice (see also Kuhlmann, this volume). Here, the perceived failure of the statutory organisations, especially in terms of containing costs, provides important leverage for change. The governance of medical performance therefore consists of strong elements of network-like governing in the form of formal negotiations, which are combined with hierarchy and professional self-regulation.

Pathways of governing medical performance

The institutional contexts of the governance of medical performance across our countries are characterised by considerable diversity on all three dimensions, as Table 2.1 illustrates. The variations among the entrenched command-and-control healthcare states are particularly interesting. In Britain and Norway the type of healthcare state coincides with a considerable degree of centralisation of governing arrangements, whereas Denmark is characterised by greater decentralisation. The diversity is even greater in relation to the normative institutions related to the private interest government of doctors. In Denmark and Norway medical authority is very firmly embedded and connected to the predominantly public governance of healthcare. This contrasts with Britain, which is a classic example of where medical authority is first and foremost based on professional self-regulation. In between those two extremes are Italy and Germany.

Having looked at the institutional contexts, what are the corresponding pathways of governing medical performance? Table 2.2 provides an overview. Professional self-regulation is present in countries reflecting an especially strong

Table 2.2: Pathways of the governance of medical performance

	Britain	Italy	Denmark	Norway	Germany
Mode(s) of governance	Hierarchy; separate professional self-regulation	Professional self-regulation; some hierarchy	Hierarchy; network; some market/ competition	Hierarchy; network	Professional self-regulation; some network; some hierarchy

legacy of medical dominance in this area of governance, although in a more covert form in Denmark and Norway. However, professional self-regulation exists side by side with other forms of governance, as doctors are part of public systems of providing healthcare. Importantly, countries vary in terms of the relative balance between different forms of governance and this points to the respective institutions at play here. In Britain as well as in Denmark and Norway hierarchy is key, which in many ways resonates with the thrust of the command-and-control healthcare state. Hierarchy is less strong in Italy, reflecting the weakness of the state in healthcare typical of insecure command-and-control healthcare states. This is exacerbated by the considerable degree of decentralisation of governance arrangements together with the fact that medical authority is weakly embedded in public contexts and instead based on private practice. Hierarchy is also weaker in Germany, although for a different set of reasons, notably the close association between joint self-administration as a form of network-based governing with professional self-regulation. This corresponds to a form of medical authority that is highly institutionalised. However, as Denmark and Norway demonstrate, hierarchy and network-based forms of governing are not necessarily exclusive. On the contrary, consensus-oriented negotiations are part and parcel of hierarchically oriented governing here. At institutional level, this is based, among other things, in a form of medical authority that is firmly embedded in the public governance of healthcare.

The institutional variations across countries are also reflected in differences related to individual forms of governing. For example, in relation to professional self-regulation, countries vary in the extent to which this form of governance is integrated into other forms of governance. The variations among the countries are particularly closely related to the normative institutions of doctors' private interest government. The 'pure' form in Britain reflects the fact that professional self-regulation provides the normative basis for medical authority. This particularly contrasts with Denmark and Norway where a highly mixed form of professional self-regulation reflects a form of medical authority that is firmly embedded in and connected to the broader public governance of healthcare. Germany and Italy assume a middle-order position.

Besides professional self-regulation in the form of indirect governing through education and dealing with cases of malpractice, negotiations also play an important role in the governance of medical performance. Negotiations tend to be associated with network-based governance, but in all our countries negotiations are more or less closely tied to hierarchical forms of governing. This in turn shapes the nature of negotiations. The relationship with hierarchy is particularly strong in Germany, making for highly institutionalised negotiations. This applies to a lesser extent to Denmark and Norway, where negotiations are formal by virtue of being part of the healthcare state. This is different in Italy and also in Britain, where negotiations are informal and exist side by side with hierarchy-based governance.

Finally, the nature of hierarchy-based governance also varies among the countries, especially reflecting the relative (de)centralisation of power in governing arrangements. In Britain, hierarchical governing is highly centralised, whereas in Italy, Denmark and Germany hierarchical governing is more decentralised and closely tied with negotiations. As such, negotiations as a form of network-based governance emerge as an important mediator between professional self-regulation and hierarchy-based forms of governance. This is also reflected in differences in the normative institutions of medical governance in our countries. For example, whereas Denmark and Norway appear to be dominated by cooperative and integrative norms concerning the relationship between doctors and the state, the relationship between doctors and the state in Britain and Italy is more based on detachment and confrontation.

The new governance of medical performance

The analysis above presents the governance of medical performance as a combination of different logics, with professional self-regulation co-existing (more or less closely) with other forms of governing. There are two things that are changing with the 'new' governance of medical performance. First, the relationship between professional self-regulation and other forms of governing is coming to the fore. Hierarchy is thus not losing ground, instead it is reinventing its role as an active regulator using new combinations of control, incentives for self-governance, and interaction in networks across formal government levels, as well as the public and private sectors. Second, this also makes for a more explicit regime of governing medical performance. What are the specific characteristics of the new governance of medical performance in individual countries? And, in what ways do these characteristics reflect the respective institutional contexts and associated paths discussed above?

In Britain, the new governance of medical performance emerges as two separate sets of governing mechanisms centring on clinical governance and revalidation respectively. This reflects the fact that private interest government is quite separate from the rest of the healthcare state. Interestingly, the emerging competition between the two sets of governing mechanisms provides leverage for change, as reflected in the discussion about the possible integration of governing mechanisms. The fact that collectively the medical profession has not fully succeeded in adapting its strategies to the policy challenges potentially contributes to this process. Here it is indicative that the interests of the medical organisations have often remained fragmented, reflecting growing divisions between rank and file. The implications for the governance of medical performance are twofold: the strengthening of hierarchy-based governance, notably through the introduction of clinical governance; and the addition of network-based governance (in the form of negotiations among medical organisations) to traditionally exclusively professional self-regulation. The first set of developments has been characterised by hectic institution building, although the effect on the workings of medical governance remains uncertain (Salter, 2004).

In contrast, in Italy the new governance of medical performance presents itself as a more unified approach (Tousijn, 2005). The 'management by objectives' reflects the increasing importance of regional, decentralised public management within healthcare. Here, the tensions within the institutions of the governance of consumption and provision, especially between the central and local levels and between public and private elements, have provided leverage for change. Importantly, change remains incomplete and it is indicative that informal negotiations as a form of network-based governance complement hierarchical management by objectives. In fact, besides the introduction of hierarchy-based governance, this is the main aspect of the new governance of medical performance.

In Denmark and Norway decentralised public management also provides the platform for the new governance of medical performance. Contracts between counties and hospitals, together with clinical governance in Denmark and the introduction of general management in hospitals in addition to patient lists for GPs in Norway, point to a more hierarchical and above all centralised approach to governing medical performance. In contrast to Italy, but also Britain, the changes are also more incremental, at least in the Danish case (Pedersen et al, 2005; Vrangbæk and Christiansen, 2005). Possible explanations are that the structures of public management are not only decentralised as in Italy (although this applies to a lesser extent to Norway), but also embedded in a system of formal negotiations and consensus seeking. The development of reform initiatives often also occurs from the bottom up (Vrangbæk and Martinsen, 2005). Further, the tight integration of private interest government into institutions for the governance of consumption and provision makes the emergence of a separate strategy based on professional self-regulation as in Britain unlikely. Underlining the embeddedness of professions in the state, the historical development of the central Norwegian health administration has been seen as an 'extension of the medical clinic into the state' (Byrkjeflot, 2004, p 56; Nordby, 1989).

In Germany, by contrast, the institutions of the (partly joint) self-administration of insurance funds and doctors, together with underlying tensions – especially relating to issues of financial control – provide the main platform for change (for an overview see Urban, 2001; Di Luzio, 2004; Rosenbrock and Gerlinger, 2004). Here, the new governance of medical performance consists of a wide range of initiatives that are concerned with extending the scope of existing governing arrangements and with changing the underlying logic(s) of governance. This includes altering the balance between professional self-regulation on the one hand and network, and hierarchy-based governance on the other, as well as strengthening the hierarchical elements of joint self-administration. As in Denmark and Norway and in contrast to Britain, and to some extent Italy, change tends to be incremental, not least reflecting the strength of formal negotiations that also involve doctors. This is particularly true in the case of medical performance that has traditionally been the territory of doctors.

Comparing the old and new governance of medical performance

The comparative analysis above suggests a number of things about the new governance of medical performance (see Table 2.3 for an overview). The developments in all countries point to the emergence of a more explicit regime of governance and hierarchy-based forms of governing are gaining ground. In all countries except Italy the strengthening of hierarchy has coincided with a centralisation of power in governing arrangements. This is particularly significant in relation to Germany, Denmark and Norway with healthcare states that have traditionally been more decentralised.

The prominence of hierarchy in the new governance of medical performance in all five countries is interesting considering the significant differences in institutional contexts and associated pathways of governing medical performance. However, differences do come to the fore when looking more closely at the specific nature of hierarchy and the specific ways in which hierarchy is combined with other forms of governing. Here, interesting variations emerge: Britain is characterised by more (centralised) hierarchy with parallel, professional self-regulation; in Italy incomplete (regional) hierarchy is combined with informal negotiations; whereas in Denmark, Norway and Germany more and increasingly centralised hierarchy is intertwined with formal negotiations, although the focus of negotiations varies. These variations point to differences in existing pathways of the governance of medical performance and the respective institutional contexts.

In Britain, for example, a strongly centralised command-and-control healthcare state provides a platform for the considerable strengthening of hierarchical governing. Yet, combined with normative institutions that perceive medical authority as first and foremost based on professional self-regulation, this leads

Table 2.3: Old/new pathways of governing medical performance

Pathways	Britain	Italy	Denmark	Norway	Germany
Old governance of medical performance	Hierarchy; separate professional self-regulation	Professional self-regulation; some hierarchy	Hierarchy; network	Hierarchy; network	Professional self-regulation; some network; some hierarchy
New governance of medical performance	More hierarchy; a lot of market; competition between regimes	More hierarchy; some market; some network	More hierarchy; some market	More hierarchy; some market	More network; more hierarchy; some market

to the emergence of a parallel regime of governance. A similar friction exists in Italy, but for different reasons. Here, a hierarchical approach to governing in the form of new public management has been implanted on an insecure and highly decentralised healthcare state, as well as a form of medical authority that is first and foremost based on private practice. This makes not only for incomplete hierarchy, but also gives primary place to informal negotiations. In contrast, in Germany hierarchy takes the form of circumscribing, in an increasingly tighter way, joint self-administration as a form of network-based governing. This reflects the strength of the legacy of formal negotiations between doctors and insurance funds.

In addition, in all countries elements of market- (competition-)based governance have been introduced, taking the form of patient choice, competitive contracting and activity-based payment – albeit in varying institutional forms and within more or less tightly controlled frameworks. Although there probably has always existed some type of informal benchmarking and ranking, the new feature of current developments is the strong emphasis on formalisation and the explicit link to economic incentives. Importantly, however, the impact of specific institutional contexts is also visible here. Compared to other countries Britain is characterised by an extensive set of market mechanisms. This points to the close association between markets and hierarchy: strong markets are predicated upon strong hierarchies (Freeman, 1998). It is precisely these forms of hierarchical governing, coupled with a high degree of centralisation, that are especially strong in the case of Britain.

Institutions and pathways of change revisited

The chapter began by noting that the market has been central to reforms across many countries, as evidenced by the prominence of managed competition. At the same time, experiences with markets in healthcare suggest that the reforms not only have included considerable re-regulation, but that such re-regulation also remains firmly embedded in country-specific contexts. Based on a case study of the governance of medical performance, the analysis suggests two things.

First, the developments in all five countries point to the fact that the new medical governance is indeed characterised by strong elements of hierarchy-based forms of governance, but ones that are combined with other modes of governing, often in the form of hybrids. This means that old and new forms of governing exist side by side and even strongly interact with each other. The situation is further complicated by the importance of horizontal and vertical decentralisation in relation to decisions about the governance of medical performance. The sector-specific institutions of healthcare are characterised by more or less strong elements of vertical decentralisation – especially Italy, Denmark and to some extent Norway. Equally, non-government actors often also play an influential role in this area of governance and here the importance of negotiations is indicative. Germany and Italy and to some degree Britain are good examples here.

Second, although the developments in the five countries share some commonalities in terms of the characteristics of the new governance of medical performance, there are important differences in relation to the specific form of governance. This applies to the relative balance between forms of governance, the specific meaning of individual forms of governing and the specific interaction between different forms of governance. Such differences point not only to conjunctural factors, but importantly also to institutional differences related to the respective healthcare state, and the degrees of (de)centralisation of governing arrangements, together with the normative institutions associated with doctors' private interest government. In terms of the balance between different forms of governance, for example, the type of healthcare state impacts on the relative strength of hierarchy in the new governance of medical performance. Here, Britain and Italy are at opposite ends of the spectrum. In the case of Britain, the combination of an entrenched command-and-control healthcare state with highly centralised governing arrangements gives primacy to hierarchy-based forms of governing. Italy, by contrast, combines an insecure command-and-control healthcare state with highly decentralised governing arrangements and this means that hierarchy-based forms of governing are weaker and also co-exist with network-based forms of governing. In terms of the nature of individual forms of governing, the variations among the still strong forms of professional self-regulation are an interesting example. These vary from pure and separate forms of professional self-regulation to mixed and integrated forms.

This points to differences relating to the underlying normative institutions of doctors' private interest government: medical authority based on professional self-regulation in Britain makes for pureness and separateness, while more embedded forms of medical authority such as in Denmark and Norway, but to some extent also Germany, make for more integrated/institutionalised forms of professional self-regulation. This example also highlights the institutional embeddedness of the interplay between different forms of governance. In sum, understanding institutions therefore holds the key to identifying and explaining pathways of change.

Note

[1] This chapter is part of an international research project entitled 'Governing Doctors: A Comparative Analysis of Pathways of Change', funded by the Danish Social Science Research Council. The aim of the project is to identify and explain the country-specific pathways of change in the governing of doctors in four countries: Denmark, Germany, Italy and the UK. The inclusion of Norway is part of a parallel research collaboration with Simon Neby at the Stein Rokkan Center at the University of Bergen. We are grateful to our colleagues Brian Salter, Simon Neby and Willem Tousijn for allowing us to use material from their country reports and for providing comments on earlier versions of this chapter.

References

Burau, V. (2005) 'Comparing professions through actor-centred governance: community nursing in Britain and Germany', *Sociology of Health and Illness*, vol 27, no 1, pp 114-37.

Busse, R. and Riesberg, A. (2004) *Health care systems in transition: Germany*, Copenhagen: WHO Regional Office for Europe on behalf of the European Observatory on Health Systems and Policies.

Byrkjeflot, H. (2004) 'The making of a health care state? An analysis of the recent hospital reform in Norway', in A. Andresen, T. Grønlie and S.A. Skålevåg (eds) *Hospitals, patients and medicine 1800–2000*, Report 6-2004, Bergen: The Stein Rokkan Centre for Social Studies.

Byrkjeflot, H. and Neby, S. (2004) 'The decentralized path challenged? Nordic health care reforms in comparison', Working Paper 2-2004, Bergen: The Stein Rokkan Centre for Social Studies.

Di Luzio, G. (2004) 'The irresistible decline of the medical profession? An empirical investigation of its autonomy and economic situation in the changing German welfare state', *German Politics*, vol 13, no 3, pp 419-48.

Freeman, R. (1998) 'The Germany model: the state and the market in health care', in W. Ranade (ed) *Markets and health care: A comparative analysis*, London: Longman, pp 179-93.

Grytten, J., Skau, I., Sørensen, R.J. and Aasland, O.G. (2003) *Fastlegereformen: En analyse av fastlegenes arbeidsbelastning og tjenestetilbud*, Forskningsrapport 11/2003, Sandvika, Handelshøyskolen BI.

Irvine, D. (2003) *The doctor's tale: Professionalism and public trust*, Oxford: Radcliffe Medical Press.

March, J.G. and Olsen, J.P. (1989) *Rediscovering institutions: The organizational basis of politics*, New York: Free Press.

Moran, M. (1999) *Governing the health care state: A comparative study of the United Kingdom, the United States and Germany*, Manchester: Manchester University Press.

Moran, M. (2000) 'Understanding the welfare state: the case of health care', *British Journal of Politics and International Relations*, vol 2, no 2, pp 135-60.

Newman, J. (2001) *Modernising governance: New Labour, policy and society*, London: Sage Publications.

Nolte, E., McKee, M. and Wait, S. (2005) 'Describing and evaluating health systems', in A. Bowling and S. Ebrahim (eds) *Handbook of health research methods*, Maidenhead: Open University.

Nordby, T. (1989) *Karl Evang: En Biografi*, Oslo: Aschehoug.

Pedersen, K.M. (2005) *Sundhedspolitik: Beslutningsgrundlag, beslutningstagen og beslutninger i sundhedsvæsenet*, Odense: Syddansk Universitetsforlag.

Pedersen, K.M., Beck, M. and Christiansen, T. (2005) 'The Danish health care system: evolution – not revolution – in a decentralized system', *Health Economics*, vol 14, no 1, pp 41-57.

Rosenbrock, R. and Gerlinger, T. (2004) *Gesundheitspolitik: Eine systematische Einführung*, Bern: Hans Huber.

Salter, B. (2001) 'Who rules? The new politics of medical regulation', *Social Science and Medicine*, vol 52, pp 871-83.

Salter, B. (2004) *The new politics of medicine*, Basingstoke: Palgrave Macmillan.

Tousijn, W. (2005) 'Country report: Italy', Unpublished manuscript.

Urban, H.J. (2001) *Wettbewerbskorporatistische Regulierung im Politikfeld Gesundheit: Der Bundesausschuss der Ärzte und Krankenkassen und die gesundheitspolitische Wende*, WZB Discussion Paper, P01-206, Berlin: Wissenschaftszentrum Berlin für Sozialforschung.

Vrangbæk, K. and Christiansen, T. (2005) 'Health policy in Denmark: leaving the decentralized welfare path?', *Journal of Health Politics, Policy and Law*, vol 30, no 1-2, pp 29-52.

Vrangbæk, K. and Martinsen, D.S. (2005) 'Sporskifte i dansk sundhedspolitik', *Økonomi & Politik*, vol 78, no 1, pp 18-30.

THREE

Governing beyond markets and managerialism: professions as mediators[1]

Ellen Kuhlmann

Introduction

Across countries healthcare systems respond to new needs and demands with the introduction of marketisation and new public management regimes, including a number of performance indicators and benchmarks operating at a meso level of professional governance as well as improved user participation both in the policy process and clinical decision making. These strategies bring about greater control of providers and enhance transformations towards more demand-led services. There is still much controversy, however, especially over the benefits of professional self-regulation and the options of new governance to shift the balance of power away from the medical profession (Davies, 2006; Gabe et al, 2006).

This chapter attempts to highlight the transformability of the 'private interest government' (Moran, 1999) of professions and how it is targeted by institutional pathways of changing professional governance. It brings into view the linkage between policy and professionalism and a potential for modernising health systems. This approach moves beyond the controversies of marketisation/bureaucratic regulation, and the submergence/convergence of health systems and focuses instead on the role of the professions as 'mediators' between the state and its citizens.

The German health system serves as a case study to assess the dynamics of health reform in a non-Anglo-American context, and to explore a nation-specific set of policy drivers. Empirical material comprises document analysis, a questionnaire study of physicians and qualitative data on physicians, physiotherapists and surgery receptionists (Kuhlmann, 2006). While Bismarckian social policy, especially healthcare, epitomised models of social security and justice for about a century, nowadays a corporatist structure is viewed as a barrier to innovation. At the same time, elements of corporatism and professional self-regulation allow for flexibility and responsiveness and may 'buffer' social conflict (Stacey, 1992); they are even gaining ground in state-centred health systems (Hunter, 2006). Germany thus provides an interesting example to study both the weaknesses and benefits of professional self-regulation and how they interface with institutional contexts.

The chapter starts with an outline of a dynamic approach to the relationships between professions, the state and the public. This is followed by an exploration of a country-specific pattern of policy drivers and how it is linked to changing patterns of professionalism. Finally, some conclusions are drawn on the embeddedness of medical power and an innovative potential of professionalisation that may contribute to the demands on 'accountability' of professions and a more integrated health workforce.

Professions as mediators: linking modernisation and professionalisation

Change in healthcare is driven by various forces, which cannot be assessed by simply looking at health policy and institutional regulation. Economic constraints, together with workforce changes – including shifts in gender arrangements – and new demands on social inclusion and participation call for a new balance between professional independence and public control. Combining theories of governance with theoretical concepts from the sociology of professions helps to analyse the changes under way within a broader framework of societal change and the processes of modernisation.

Following Newman (2005), governance includes social and cultural as well as institutional practices. The author argues that changing governance is not simply the result of pressure, whether from above or below. Instead, it embodies a 'remaking of people, politics and public spheres', and complex dynamics rather than a uniform trend (Newman, 2005; see also Clarke, 2004). From this perspective, professionalism and the 'private interest government' of the medical profession (Moran, 1999) are specific governance practices that intersect with other forms of governance (see also Burau and Vrangbæk, this volume).

From an historical point of view the rise of professionalism and the emergence of professional projects are characteristic of civic societies (Bertilsson, 1990). Professions continue to play a pivotal role in the concepts of welfare states and their transformation to service-driven societies, which are characterised, on the whole, by an expansion of expert knowledge and professionalism. Moran (2004, p 31) argues that 'the welfare state was a professional state; it depended on professionals both for the expertise needed to formulate policy and to deliver that policy'. This statement underscores the interdependence of professions, the state and the public.

Following Bertilsson (1990, p 131) one can 'work out the negotiable status of our social citizenship by means of an interest theory of the professions'. The developing welfare states had a vital interest in the expansion of professional projects. As they promised access to social services for the citizens, they had to provide and expand the markets for professionalised work. From the public's perspective these services offered by the professions became a gauge for the success of the attempts of welfare states to translate the concept of social citizenship into the practice of social services. Professionalism also serves as an ideological model for 'justifying inequality of status and closure of access in the occupational order' (Larson, 1977, p xviii). The state made use of professionalism, both as a strategy for participation in the 'merits' of civic society and as a strategy to legitimise exclusion. In this latter sense, professionalism and the self-regulatory bodies can serve to reduce social conflicts. Self-regulation is assumed to be more effective and 'to produce higher levels of trust between the regulated and the regulatory bodies than in the case with direct regulation', and it also saves cost (Baggott, 2002, p 34).

However, state regulation is undergoing fundamental changes in all areas of public services. In healthcare, new public management and forms of open coordination and network governance are signs of an ongoing development towards the 're-shaping of the state from above, from within, from below' (Reich, 2002, p 1669; see Burau, 2005; Radcliff and Dent, 2005). Medical – or 'clinical' – governance plays a key role within these scenarios of change towards more demand-led and user-friendly health systems; evidence-based medicine and decision making pervade all areas of healthcare and health policy (Gray and Harrison, 2004). A new pattern of 'technogovernance' (May et al, 2006) is accompanied by a changing role of the service user (Allsop et al, 2004; Clarke et al, 2007; Newman and Kuhlmann, 2007).

At the same time, there are also ongoing transformations on the provider side. Professionalism is becoming more diverse and context dependent; and new professional projects are springing up that apply new strategies to professionalisation issues. Across Europe, and even beyond, a new need to 'govern at a distance' (Miller and Rose, 1990) and to bridge the interests of different stakeholders – including nation states – creates a new demand for the legitimatory power of professional knowledge practices and public trust in welfare state services. There is increasing evidence of a 'new' professionalism, which is significantly different from earlier forms. Although the traditional exclusionary tactics of the professions have not yet been overcome, professionalism is not necessarily a barrier to modernisation; it also carries the potential for innovation in healthcare.

Professions may counteract the state and the market in the sense of a 'third logic' (Freidson, 2001; see Kremer and Tonkens, 2006). The professions may be champions of the 'people', especially patients, thus following an 'altruistic mission' and a 'public interest' (Saks, 1995), and they may also exercise their 'private interest government' (Moran, 1999). The double role of professions as 'officers' and 'servants' of the public embodies a number of ambiguities and uncertainties. These classic ambiguities nowadays meet with the 'unsettled formations of welfare, state and nation', as Clarke (2004, p 25) terms it. Accordingly, the triangle set out in Figure 3.1 comprising health professions, the state and the public must be understood as dynamic relationships that allow for various ways to model and remodel power relations in healthcare systems.

Within the scope of governance of changing welfare states, the professionals are needed – perhaps more than ever – to legitimise political decisions and to maintain public trust in social services, especially in view of leaner budgets and more demanding service users. In this sense, the biomedical knowledge system

Figure 3.1: Professions, the state and the public: dynamic relationships

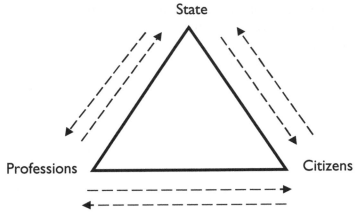

Source: Kuhlmann (2006, p 225)

is the most powerful governance practice and doctors the most trusted group in society, although changes are under way in both areas (see also Calnan and Rowe, this volume).

The 'remaking of governance' (Newman, 2005) and the rise of new patterns of professionalism are two sides of the same coin, namely the modernisation of welfare states driven by 'global' forces and strategies on one side, but shaped by national regulatory frameworks on the other. The following sections explore the linkage between policy and actor-based changes in the professions.

Remodelling a corporatist health system: change and conservative forces

Germany does not fit into the typology of either market-driven or state-centred restructuring; it has its one strong and longlasting tradition of social policy, and the longest tradition of compulsory social health. The health system is based on corporatism, federalism and decentralisation of power (for an overview see Moran, 1999; Rosenbrock and Gerlinger, 2006). As a rule, Statutory Health Insurance (SHI), which covers 90% of the population, is financed jointly by employers and employees. Regulation is based on two pillars: the SHI funds that represent the purchaser and the user side, and the self-governing bodies of the medical profession that represent the provider side. Those outside the medical professions are denied the status of a profession and excluded from the regulatory bodies (except psychotherapists who are partly integrated in the professional bodies of medicine). Although regulatory bodies have recently been expanded and market logic, together with a more interventionist role of the state, is gaining ground, the corporatist model of delegating power to doctors and sickness funds as the two pillars of SHI care remains strong.

Striking advantages of compulsory health insurance for all citizens – easy access to health services, and the solidarity and responsiveness of the Bismarckian system – go hand in hand with fundamental weaknesses of the system. A major critique focuses on the high fragmentation of providers and services combined with an orthodox curative orientation and a physician-centred system. Recent reviews from the Advisory Council (SVR, 2003, 2005) highlight the need to improve the coordination of provider services, quality management and user participation. A series of reform Acts from the 1990s onwards bears witness to strong pressure to innovate as far as the health system is concerned.

Despite a wide range of system weaknesses, cost containment is the most powerful policy driver for change. The US strategy of cost control – managed competition – was used to point the way to restructuring. The introduction of a free choice of sickness funds for all citizens and market competition within the SHI system, legally fixed budgets on the provider side, the exclusion of several health services from SHI care and increasing co-payment of patients bear witness to this driver, which was strengthened as the 1990s progressed. Marketisation and the dominance of cost containment reflect a 'global turn' towards neoliberalism in healthcare systems. However, since the beginning of the 21st century, patterns from new public management and state regulation have been gaining ground and policy goals extended (Glaeske et al, 2001; SVR, 2003, 2005).

Characteristic of new policies is that they are directed primarily at a short-term reduction of costs and addressed almost exclusively to the medical profession and the SHI funds (see for instance, Greß et al, 2006; Stuck et al, 2007). The politics of cost containment fail to address the key problem of the health economy, namely the falling income rate and demographic change. They also fail to respond to the wide range of new demands, and do not systematically touch on the system deficits of healthcare. Various attempts to further organisational change have largely failed, and no comprehensive system of public control of providers and quality of care has so far been established (SVR, 2003). At the same time, the politics of marketisation enhanced change in the system of SHI funds, in particular a growing merger of funds and a move away from bureaucratic towards more flexible and service-oriented organisations (Bode, 2003). However, these developments also provoked unintended dynamics in the SHI system, for instance growing social inequality due to the increased co-payment of users and the exclusion of certain services from SHI care, and increased pressure on physicians to act in accordance with financial interests.

While it is true that the reform Acts were less successful than some had hoped, they nevertheless opened the way for other important changes and future prospects. Health policy is increasingly turning to individual providers – instead of the hitherto collective contracts with the SHI physicians' associations – and expanding their options with regard to contracting and provider organisation (Di Luzio, 2004). This strategy provides new resources to shift the balance of power away from the physicians' associations and to engage SHI funds in the key priorities of the state. This reflects a salient interest of the state that is as old as Statutory Health itself.

The strengthening of SHI funds was especially pronounced in times of economic crisis, like the Weimar Republic, and lost ground in the 'golden age' of medicine in the post-war period. Given problems in the 21st century of cost containment in the healthcare system, the strategy is facing revival once again.

The reform Acts confirm that a classic pattern of solving financial problems by simply shifting the balance of power within the stakeholder arrangement continues to dominate health policy. At the same time, policy goals are becoming more diverse, particularly in their reflection of a need for quality management, new models of care and user participation. Rather than a 'decorporatisation' Germany faces various transformations of corporatism enhanced through patterns drawn from new governance. One important arena is the organisation of care where the transformations can be observed 'in action'.

Advancing organisational change

Change in the organisation of providers becomes a 'global' strategy to catch up with arrears in the modernisation of health systems and establish integrated caring models. In imitation of reform models introduced in the industrial sector, concepts of teamwork that embody multidisciplinary qualifications, cooperative working arrangements and flat hierarchies are the preferred strategy in the health sector (McKee et al, 2006; Maynard and Street, 2006). International research reveals that key conditions of effective integrated caring models are the collaboration of the diverse occupational groups involved, formalised work arrangements, quality management and a cooperative organisational culture. Strong barriers to integration are medical dominance and 'tribalism' in healthcare, but also a lack of standards and formalisation of work (Richards et al, 2000; McKee et al, 2006). Organisations have thus become the veritable 'switchboards' of changing health systems.

Precisely in these areas, regulation in Germany is weakest and focuses on the medical profession. The German version of integrated care comes in the form of the 'cooperation of physicians' and 'medical provider networks', as the various pilot projects bring to the fore (Di Luzio, 2004). This is in stark contrast to the global models of restructuring that include a wider range of occupational groups, and impact more directly on the organisational level. In Germany, neither Managed Care Organisations (MCOs), like those established in the US (Donaldson et al, 1996), nor a state regulated merger of physicians, as introduced in Britain (Fulop et al, 2005), are fostered. Although health policy is attempting to shift the balance of power towards the SHI funds, the options are markedly different from those that exist for MCO managers or within the National Health Service. SHI funds do not have the power to directly intervene on the organisational level as long as physicians' associations have the monopoly on the provision of ambulatory care.

While this powerful position is on the wane, organisational change remains a result of negotiations between SHI funds and physicians; and an outcome of managerial change cannot be taken for granted. Consequently, SHI interventions are generally limited. Health policy – and SHI funds – provides financial incentives, while the process of merging providers of healthcare into networks and medical centres is currently controlled by the medical profession. Future options and the success of SHI funds in targeting provider networks are hardly predictable. Added to this, there are currently no signs that SHI funds systematically include the health occupations in new merger policies.

The attempts to shift the balance of power from in-patient to ambulatory care and from specialists to generalists in health policy are in line with international developments. Nevertheless, the German version of integrated care differs significantly from the models of primary care developed in Anglo-American health systems (see for instance Donaldson et al, 1996; Tovey and Adams, 2001). Essential regulatory elements of the latter, such as limited access to specialists and the concomitant gatekeeper function of generalists, have not yet been successfully introduced in Germany. Most importantly, these models contradict patients' right to choose a doctor, and more generally, infringe the legal rules and a culture of citizen rights that grant access to an entire spectrum of services covered by SHI care. Over and above this, new organisational models in Germany are shaped by the deficits of a classic pattern of corporatist regulation that focuses on the medical profession.

The corporatist system allows for high flexibility. It provides a number of options both to enhance cooperation between providers, but also to outflank policy incentives towards integrated care. Under these conditions, options for change in the organisation of healthcare are more individualised and dependent on institutional environments and organisational context. Consequently, the outcome is less stable and predictable, and this in turn creates a new need for negotiations. The crucial issue is that the most powerful actors – in particular the medical profession – have better resources at their disposal to promote their interests than new players, like the various other health occupations.

Drivers for change and national pathways of corporatism

A global discourse of restructuring is being taken up in Germany that attempts to strengthen ambulatory care and general medicine, prevention and user involvement. The regulatory system and the biomedical approach have both been extended, but the corporatist structure is not replaced by new patterns. This is most evident in the new programmes for chronic illness, called disease management programmes (DMPs) (SVR, 2005; Greß et al, 2006). The DMPs focus, for the first time, on organisational change and tighter control of physicians; the aim is to improve standardisation and transparency of healthcare services by target setting, performance indicators and mandatory evaluations. However, health policy's move towards new governance is shaped by a classic pattern of corporatist regulation based on two key actors and by the politics of cost containment. The government reinforces efforts to engage the SHI funds in its key goals but largely ignores other health occupations; the role of the users of healthcare services also remains weak and no comprehensive system of public control has yet been established. This marks an important difference from the strategies applied in Anglo-American countries, where the stakeholder arrangement is increasingly becoming more diverse and public control is reinforced (see Allsop and Jones, this volume).

To a certain degree, Germany's health system reflects international developments, but the corporatist tradition does not simply give way to global models of reform. Nonetheless, the historical monoliths of SHI funds and the medical profession are becoming permeable and more open to new actors. A new willingness of the government to widen the circle of players involved in regulation challenges the corporatist 'giants' – the SHI funds and physicians' associations – and may pave the way for further changes, like inclusion of new players from the health occupations. These developments may provoke fissures in the seemingly stable arrangement of physicians and SHI funds. The process of change is not simply slower in Germany, but different from Anglo-American countries. The question must especially be addressed as to whether the strong stakeholder position of the medical profession in Germany and the lack of a comprehensive coordination of services provided by other health occupations actually allows for the broadening of the range of providers of care and the epistemological basis of that care.

Figure 3.2 summarises the main drivers for change, differntiating between strong and weak drivers. A review of the literature suggests that a primary care approach and a regulatory system that includes a broad range of health professional groups are the strongest drivers for change in the organisation and provision of care. More explicit interventions at the organisational level – for instance, the merger of providers into networks and trusts – and the establishment of a complex system of public control also increase the amount of significant change. Compared to this, consumerism and the various forms of managerial control appear as weaker drivers for change in healthcare (Kuhlmann, 2006).

Characteristic of health policy in Germany is that it advances the weaker drivers more than the stronger ones. The tide is nevertheless turning towards intervention in the organisation of care and thus towards a stronger driver for modernisation. Neglecting strong drivers for change on the level of institutional regulation has considerable consequences for modernisation processes on the meso and micro levels. This negligence impacts on the organisation of care and limits the options for change. The other side of this coin represents new opportunities for the professions to fill the emerging voids in the governing of organisational change and cooperation between providers. This pattern of governance allows those involved in the negotiations to define and redefine the indicators and methods of managerialism, and the strategies to improve cooperation of providers. Owing to the powerful position of physicians and a lack of state support for the health occupations, the medical profession has the strongest resources to successfully use the new opportunities. The lack of comprehensive state regulation and acknowledgement of the health occupations in Germany as professions represents a major obstacle to the realisation of integrated caring models and interprofessional cooperation.

Figure 3.2: Strong and weak drivers for change

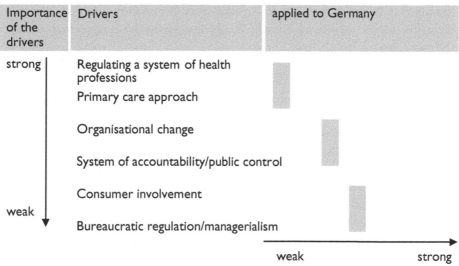

Importance of the drivers	Drivers	applied to Germany
strong	Regulating a system of health professions	
	Primary care approach	
	Organisational change	
	System of accountability/public control	
	Consumer involvement	
weak	Bureaucratic regulation/managerialism	

weak   strong

Source: Kuhlmann (2006, p 95)

Professionalism revisited: conservative and more inclusive elements

Professions do not simply react to health policy – they can also enhance change. A consequence of weak state regulation is that a variety of regulatory mechanisms and change emerging from the health workforce bottom up become more important. In this situation, interest-based strategies of the health occupations and the medical profession follow new pathways that are not fully under the control of the government. Although each group is in the process of renegotiating its place in the health system, the medical profession has the greatest ability to flexibly combine classic and new patterns of professionalism, and to develop new strategies.

The findings of my study reveal the following picture: the medical profession – commonly viewed as a conservative actor – takes up and transforms elements from new governance aimed at controlling providers into successful strategies to promote its own professional interests. The key areas where changes are manifest include quality management, coordination of provider services and patient information (see also Di Luzio, 2004). The emergence of managerialism, networks and more contextualised identities indicates that changes are under way in the structure, action and culture of the medical profession.

Physicians feel a need to overcome 'encrusted' patterns of SHI regulation and 'stiff grandfathers' and 'bureaucrats' even in the profession's own bodies, as some participants in my study expressed it. They are calling for the modernisation of medical self-regulation from the bottom up. However, they do not aim to replace corporatist institutions. Rather, the improvement of coordination through networks and more participatory bottom-up structures of decision making release dynamics into the governance process, the organisation of healthcare and the health workforce that may contribute to modernisation processes and social inclusion. Consequently, professions do not necessarily act as conservative forces; they can also enable change.

The rise of new patterns of professionalism is equally striking with regard to the health occupations included in the study who occupy different positions in the health workforce: physiotherapists represent a middle-range occupation with advanced professionalisation, academic training and increasing proportions of men (approximately 20%). By contrast, surgery receptionists are a 99% female group positioned at the very bottom of the health workforce. In 2006, following European standards, efforts to improve the status of this occupation were partly successful and these healthcare workers were renamed physicians' assistants. For both occupational groups, classic strategies aimed at advancing the transformation of an occupational group into a profession are not available, especially state protection and market closure. Moreover, the health occupations apply hybrid strategies based on various elements of professionalism and individualised tactics linked to market power. However, the slow pace of professionalisation of health occupations in Germany underscores the limitations of such tactics. On top of this, there is a lack of collective strategies aimed at inclusion in the legal framework of SHI regulation.

The agency of health occupations is restricted by a range of conservative forces. In particular, the strategies mirror gendered tactics of professionalisation that focus on change in the workplace and 'credentialism' rather than legalist tactics; however, credentialist tactics are generally less successful than the legalist kind (Witz, 1992). We cannot understand change in the health workforce and the regulatory frameworks without taking gender into account. Neither of the occupational groups mentioned here can effectively make use of the new opportunities provided by a policy discourse of integrated care and cooperation. Health reform in Germany turns out to be neither a facilitator in the professionalisation of physiotherapy nor a 'job machine' for surgery receptionists, although it does provide new opportunities for individuals to improve their market power. Even though the use of a discourse of professionalism is spreading to new occupational groups, this does not necessarily mean that it can be applied successfully.

Taken together, new patterns of professionalism, new strategies to promote professional interest, and new patterns of professional identity are observed in the medical profession as the archetype of a profession, as well as in occupational groups that strive for professionalisation, such as physiotherapists. At the same time, conservative forces and the exclusionary tactics of the professions continue to exist. In this situation, classic strategies of exclusion and new patterns of a more inclusive professionalism are applied simultaneously (see Table 3.1).

Exclusionary and more inclusive patterns of professionalism do not simply co-exist. They release new dynamics that lead to a greater diversity of professionalism. Existing overlaps and tensions between conflicting patterns of professionalism enhance various new forms of promoting professional interests. However, greater

Table 3.1: Diversity of professionalism between social exclusion and social inclusion

Exclusionary patterns of professionalism	More inclusive patterns of professionalism
Hierarchical, bureaucratic patterns of self-regulation and self-administration	Network governance, more active participation in the self-regulatory bodies
Striving for market closure	Cooperation and teamwork
'Tribalism' and occupational closure	Networking and more permeable occupational boundaries
Claims for 'autonomy' and self-determined decision making	Inclusion of managerialism, standardisation of care, evidence-based medicine
Quality of care based on individual qualification; 'mystique' of expert knowledge	Quality of care based on formalised procedures and performance indicators
Identity construction based on 'belonging' to a professional community	More contextualised and permeable identity constructions
Gendered division of the health workforce	Changing gender relations within professions
Expert–lay divide	Improved information, inclusion of users in regulatory bodies
Professionalism restricted to the medical and other high-status occupational groups	Various health professions refer to professionalism to upgrade occupational status

Source: Kuhlmann (2006, p 221)

diversity plays out differently in different occupational groups. Although each group is renegotiating its place in the health system, the medical profession has the greatest ability to flexibly combine classic and new patterns of professionalism, and to develop new strategies to successfully promote professional interests.

Towards diverse professional projects and more plural regulatory frameworks

This chapter has explored new options in the governance of health professionals that move beyond marketisation and managerialism. The research now reveals the rise of a 'new' professionalism that carries the seed of a more inclusive health workforce, even though it is being shaped by conservative forces. However, conservatism does not only derive from medical self-regulation. And whether the rise of a new professionalism creates 'citizen professionals' more accountable to the interests of a changing population and the public interest depends to no small degree on institutional regulatory frameworks.

One key conclusion suggested by the research is that major obstacles of modernisation do not only derive from professional politics and the hegemonic claims of the medical profession. Moreover, conservative forces are also embedded in the corporatist system and shaped by state regulation. We cannot understand the structural rigidities of the German system by simply looking at medical governance and the effects of physicians' self-regulation. In terms of the welfare state, the state is also a key actor when it comes to supporting the professionalisation of the health occupations and integrated caring models based on primary care approaches and interprofessional collaboration. In this respect medical power is fundamentally based on national configurations of state–professions relationships and a particular representation of the 'public interest'; as such, it is structurally and culturally embedded in the health system, thus creating specific pathways of change.

Another main conclusion is that the most crucial outcome of the conservatism of Germany's healthcare system is its lack of acknowledgement of the allied health professions and support workers, and their exclusion from key regulatory bodies. These deficiencies impact like a cascade on the health system and seriously limit the overall scope for reform. And, finally, professionalism and the self-governing bodies of the profession do not necessarily act as a 'countervailing power' or 'different logic' to other forms of governance, like the market and bureaucratic regulation – as suggested by some authors, especially from the US (Light, 1995; Freidson, 2001). Instead, professionalism serves as a host to different interests, strategies and identities that, in turn, may create their very own dynamics and accelerate different flows of power into the health policy process. Viewed through this lens, a greater diversity of professional projects of formerly subordinate healthcare workers and more plural regulatory bodies may counteract the hegemonic claims of the medical profession in more sustainable ways than marketisation and managerialism.

Note

[1] This chapter draws on a theoretical approach and empirical material outlined in my book *Modernising health care: Reinventing professions, the state and the public* (Kuhlmann, 2006). Here, the focus is on the institutional framing of conservative elements of professional self-regulation and the policy options for furthering a more inclusive professionalism. I am grateful to The Policy Press for allowing me to use the material.

References

Allsop, J., Jones, K. and Baggott, R. (2004) 'Health consumer groups: a new social movement?', *Sociology of Health and Illness*, vol 26, no 6, pp 737-56.

Baggott, R. (2002) 'Regulatory politics, health professionals, and the public interest', in J. Allsop and M. Saks (eds) *Regulating the health professions*, London: Routledge, pp 31-46.

Bertilsson, M. (1990) 'The welfare state, the professions and citizens', in R. Torstendahl and M. Burrage (eds) *The formation of professions: Knowledge, state and strategy*, London: Sage Publications, pp 114-33.

Bode, I. (2003) 'Multireferenzialität und Marktorientierung? Krankenkassen als hybride Organisationen im Wandel', *Zeitschrift für Soziologie*, vol 32, no 5, pp 435-53.

Burau, V. (2005) 'Comparing professions through actor-centred governance: community nursing in Britain and Germany', *Sociology of Health and Illness*, vol 27, pp 114-37.

Clarke, J. (2004) *Changing welfare, changing states: New directions in social policy*, London: Sage Publications.

Clarke, J., Newman, J., Smith, V., Vidler, E. and Westmarland, L. (2007) *Creating citizen-consumers: Changing publics, changing public services*, London, Sage Publications.

Davies, C. (2006) 'Heroes of health care? Replacing the medical profession in the policy process in the UK', in J.W. Duyvendak, T. Knijn and M. Kremer (eds) *Policy, people and the new professional*, Amsterdam: Amsterdam University Press, pp 137-51.

Di Luzio, G. (2004) 'The irresistible decline of the medical profession? An empirical investigation of its autonomy and economic situation in the changing German welfare state', *German Politics*, vol 13, pp 419-48.

Donaldson, M.S., Yordy, K.D., Lohr, K.N. and Vanselow, N.A. (1996) *Primary care: America's health in a new era*, Washington, DC: National Academy Press.

Freidson, E. (2001) *Professionalism: The third logic*, Oxford: Polity Press.

Fulop, N., Protopsalis, G., King, A., Allen, P., Hutchings, A. and Normand, C. (2005) 'Changing organisations: a study of the context and processes of mergers of health care providers in England', *Social Science and Medicine*, vol 60, pp 119-30.

Gabe, J., Kelleher, D. and Williams, G. (2006) 'Understanding medical dominance in the modern world', in D. Kelleher, J. Gabe and G. Williams (eds) *Challenging medicine* (2nd edition), London: Routledge, pp xiii-xxxiii.

Glaeske, G., Lauterbach, K.W., Rürup, B. and Wasem, J. (2001) *Weichenstellung für die Zukunft: Elemente einer neuen Gesundheitspolitik*, Berlin: Gutachten für die Friedrich-Ebert-Stiftung.

Gray, A. and Harrison, S. (eds) (2004) *Governing medicine: Theory and practice*, Milton Keynes: Open University Press.

Greß, S., Focke, A., Hessel, F. and Wasem, J. (2006) 'Financial incentives for disease management programmes and integrated care in German social health insurance', *Health Policy*, vol 78, pp 295-305.

Hunter, D.J. (2006) 'From tribalism to corporatism: the continuing managerial challenge to medical dominance', in D. Kelleher, J. Gabe and G. Williams (eds) *Challenging medicine* (2nd edition), London: Routledge, pp 1-23.

Kremer, M. and Tonkens, E. (2006) 'Authority, trust, knowledge and the public good in disarray', in J.W. Duyvendak, T. Knijn and M. Kremer (eds) *Policy, people and the new professional*, Amsterdam: Amsterdam University Press, pp 122-34.

Kuhlmann, E. (2006) *Modernising health care: Reinventing professions, the state and the public*, Bristol: The Policy Press.

Larson, M.S. (1977) *The rise of professionalism*, Berkeley, CA: University of California Press.

Light, D.W. (1995) 'Countervailing powers: a framework for professions in transition', in T. Johnson, G. Larkin and M. Saks (eds) *Health professions and the state in Europe*, London: Routledge, pp 7-24.

McKee, M., Dubois, C.-A. and Sibbard, B. (2006) 'Changing professional boundaries', in C.-A. Dubois, M. McKee and E. Nolte (eds) *Human resources for health in Europe*, Milton Keynes: Open University Press, pp 63-78.

May, C., Rapley, T., Moreira, T., Finch, T. and Heaven, B. (2006) 'Technogovernance: evidence, subjectivity, and the clinical encounter in primary care medicine', *Social Science and Medicine*, vol 62, pp 1022-30.

Maynard, A. and Street, A. (2006) 'Seven years after feast, seven years after famine: boom to bust in the NHS?', *British Medical Journal*, vol 332, pp 906-8.

Miller, P. and Rose, N. (1990) 'Governing economic life', *Economy and Society*, vol 19, no 1, pp 1-31.

Moran, M. (1999) *Governing the health care state*, Manchester: Manchester University Press.

Moran, M. (2004) 'Governing doctors in the British regulatory state', in A. Grey and S. Harrison (eds) *Medical governance: Theory and practice*, Milton Keynes: Open University Press, pp 27-36.

Newman, J. (2005) 'Introduction', in J. Newman (ed) *Remaking governance: People, politics and the public sphere*, Bristol: The Policy Press, pp 1-15.

Newman, J. and Kuhlmann, E. (2007) 'Consumers enter the political stage? Modernisation of health care in Britain and Germany', *European Journal of Social Policy*, vol 17, no 2, pp 99-111.

Radcliff, J. and Dent, M. (2005) 'Introduction: from public management to the new governance?', *Policy & Politics*, vol 33, pp 617-22.

Reich, M.R. (2002) 'Reshaping the state from above, from within, from below: implications for public health', *Social Science and Medicine*, vol 54, pp 1669-75.

Richards, A., Carley, J., Jenkins-Clarke, S. and Richards, D.A. (2000) 'Skill mix between nurses and doctors working in primary care-delegation or allocation: a review of the literature', *International Journal of Nursing Studies*, vol 37, pp 185-97.

Rosenbrock, R. and Gerlinger, T. (2006) *Gesundheitspolitik: Eine systematische Einführung* (2nd edition), Bern: Hans Huber.

Saks, M. (1995) *Professions and the public interest: Medical power, altruism and alternative medicine*, London: Routledge.

Stacey, M. (1992) *Regulating British medicine: The General Medical Council*, Chilester: Wiley.

Stuck, S.A., Redaellia, M. and Lauterbach, K.L. (2007) 'Disease management and health care reform in Germany – does more competition lead to less solidarity?', *Health Policy*, vol 80, pp 86-96.

SVR (Sachverständigenrat im Gesundheitswesen; Advisory Council for the Concerted Action in Health Care) (2003) *Health care finance, user orientation and quality*, Report summary, English version, www.svr-gesundheit.de

SVR (2005) *Koordination und Qualität im Gesundheitswesen*, Gutachten, www. svr-gesundheit.de

Tovey, P. and Adams, J. (2001) 'Primary care as intersecting social worlds', *Social Science and Medicine*, vol 52, pp 695-706.

Witz, A. (1992) *Professions and patriarchy*, London: Routledge.

FOUR

Trust relations and changing professional governance: theoretical challenges

Michael Calnan and Rosemary Rowe

Introduction

Trust is believed to be particularly salient to the provision of healthcare because it is characterised by uncertainty and an element of risk regarding the competence and intentions of the practitioner on whom the patient is reliant (Titmuss, 1968; Alaszweski, 2003). The need for interpersonal trust relates to the vulnerability associated with being ill as well as the information asymmetries and unequal relationships that arise from the specialist nature of scientific, medical knowledge. Scientific medicine's expertise, or claims to expertise, appears to be the basic condition for generating trust in this context (Rose-Ackerman, 2001) although the affective component may also have an influence (Hall et al, 2001). In the UK National Health Service (NHS), trust has traditionally played an important part in the relationship between its three key actors: the state, healthcare practitioners, and patients and the public. The post-war consensus was underpinned by trust in the 'altruistic' values associated with medical professionalism (Newman, 1998) with the state and patients tending to trust the norms of professional self-regulation and state licensing procedures to ensure that health professionals and healthcare institutions operated in the best interests of patients and citizens. Service users trusted the judgement, knowledge and expertise of health professionals to provide a competent service that met their needs and they trusted the state to ensure equity in the allocation of public goods and services.

These presumed or taken-for-granted trust relationships have, it is claimed, been challenged as a result of the introduction of changes in the organisation and funding of the health service, in the regulation and performance assessment of health professionals, and in public attitudes to healthcare and scientific medicine. This chapter seeks to explore how and why trust relations may be changing, using the NHS in the UK as a case study. It presents a theoretical framework for investigating them in future empirical research.

Definitions of trust

Trust has been characterised as a multi-layered concept primarily consisting of a cognitive element (grounded on rational and instrumental judgements) and an affective dimension (grounded on relationships and affective bonds generated through interaction, empathy and identification with others) (Mayer et al, 1995; Lewicki and Bunker, 1996; Gambetta, 1998; Gilson, 2003). Trust appears to be necessary where there is uncertainty and a level of risk, be it high, moderate or low, and this element of risk appears to be derived from an individual's uncertainty regarding the motives, intentions and future actions of another on whom the individual is dependent (Mayer et al, 1995; Mishra, 1996). Trust may vary in terms of its quality. For example, in elaborating on the nature of social capital, Putnam (2000) makes a distinction between 'thick' trust associated with close family relationships and 'thin' trust for more casual contacts.

In the context of healthcare the evidence suggests that the concept seems to embrace confidence in competence (skill and knowledge), as well as whether the trustee is working in the best interests of the trustor. The latter tends to cover honesty, confidentiality and caring, and showing respect (Mechanic and Meyer, 2000; Hall et al, 2001), whereas the former may include both technical and social/communication skills. The vulnerability associated with being ill may specifically lead trust in medical settings to have a stronger emotional and instinctive component (Coulson, 1998; Hall et al, 2001). Trust relationships are therefore traditionally characterised by one party, the trustor, having positive expectations about the competence of the other party, the trustee (competence trust), and the fact that they will work in their best interests (intentional trust). However, for some writers (Giddens, 1991) these trust relations are built on symbolic signs of expertise rather than altruistic principles and good intentions.

In the NHS we can distinguish between trust relations at the micro level between an individual patient and clinician, between one clinician and another or between a clinician and a manager, and those at the macro level, which include patient and public trust in clinicians and managers in general, in a particular healthcare organisation and in the NHS as a healthcare system (see Figure 4.1). The former are broadly categorised as interpersonal and organisational trust relations, while the latter constitute different types of institutional trust (Calnan and Rowe, 2006).

A review of the literature of trust relations in healthcare (Calnan and Rowe, 2004) highlighted that most empirical research (mainly carried out in the US) has addressed threats to patient–provider relationships and trust in healthcare systems from the patient's perspective, but studies in the organisational literature suggest that trust relations in the workforce, between providers and between providers and managers, may also influence patient–provider relationships and levels of trust. This approach suggests that trust is not primarily dispositional or an individual attribute or psychological state, but is constructed from a set of interpersonal

Figure 4.1: Framing trust relationships in healthcare

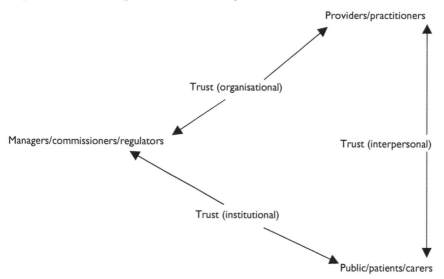

behaviours or from a shared identity. These behaviours are underpinned by sets of institutional rules, laws and customs (Gilson, 2006).

Research into trust has been conducted from a variety of disciplinary perspectives. Studies in social psychology and economics have tended to focus on the attributes of the trustor (beliefs about or calculations of trustees' motives, past experiences of healthcare and providers) and the characteristics of the trustee (their ability, competence, benevolence, integrity, reputation and communication skills). Taking the rational choice economics approach, trust may be reduced to instrumental risk assessment by individual actors – like a rational gamble that the personal gains from trusting will outweigh the risks and costs involved. For example, an economic analysis of why the public place trust in voluntary associations (Anheier and Kendall, 2002) might suggest that voluntary associations are run by those who have a stake in services provided to meet their needs and because they are non-profit making and less likely to exploit user vulnerability. However, this ignores how trust may be constructed through the use of myths, images and other symbolic constructions. Newman (1998) points to the use of informal social mechanisms, such as gossip, to communicate information through organisations, in the process contributing to the creation of trust and distrust.

The sociological literature stresses that theoretical models must also consider contextual factors: the organisational context; the stakes involved; the balance of power within the relationship; the perception of the level of risk; and the alternatives available to the trustor (Luhmann, 1979; Barber, 1983; Mayer et al, 1995; Tyler and Kramer, 1996). In this chapter we take a sociological approach seeking to understand how the meaning and enactment of trust is influenced by wider social structures and in particular how changes in the organisation and delivery of healthcare as well as broader social changes may have affected trust relations in the NHS in the UK.

Does trust matter?

The case for examining trust in healthcare tends to hinge upon theoretical arguments sometimes complemented by empirical evidence. At the level of interpersonal trust between patient and practitioner it has been argued that trust is important for its potential therapeutic effects (Mechanic, 1998), although evidence to support such claims is still in short supply mainly because of the lack of intervention studies or quasi-experimental studies examining the effect of trust on outcomes (Calnan and Rowe, 2004). However, there is a considerable body of evidence that shows that trust appears to mediate therapeutic processes and has an indirect influence on health outcomes through its impact on patient satisfaction, adherence to treatment, and continuity with a provider, and that it encourages patients to access healthcare and to make appropriate disclosure of information so that accurate and timely diagnosis can be made (Calnan and Rowe, 2004).

Trust also appears to matter to patients as well as healthcare providers. In a number of studies investigating patients' experience of healthcare, trust emerged spontaneously as a quality indicator, with patients suggesting that high-quality doctor–patient interactions are characterised by high levels of trust (for instance, Safran et al, 1998). Trust, although highly correlated with patient satisfaction (Thom and Ribisi, 1999), is believed to be a distinct concept. Trust is forward looking and reflects an attitude to a new or ongoing relationship, whereas satisfaction tends to be based on past experience and refers to assessment of providers' performance. It has been suggested that trust is a more sensitive indicator of performance than patient satisfaction (Thom et al, 2004) and might be used as a potential 'marker' for how patients evaluate the quality of healthcare.

In contrast to the sizeable literature assessing trust from the patient perspective, studies examining the value and impact of trust from the practitioner perspective and from a managerial or organisational perspective are very limited. In research that has considered the impact of trust on workplace relations in healthcare settings, trust facilitated commitment to the organisation, enhanced collaborative practice between clinicians and was associated with employee satisfaction and motivation (Gilson et al, 2005). From an organisational perspective trust is believed to be important in its own right; for instance, it is intrinsically important for the provision of effective healthcare and has even been described as a collective good, like social trust or social capital. Specific organisational benefits that might be derived from trust as a form of social capital include the reduction in transition costs due to lower surveillance and monitoring costs and the general enhancement of efficiency (Gilson, 2003).

What are the costs or dangers of trust? The abuse of power on the basis of trust is a widespread danger (Warren, 1999). As trust usually involves a relationship between trustor, trustee and a valued good, it sets up a potential power relation. Trust may provide legitimacy for the exercise of power but 'blind trust', without caution, may also enable the abuse of power, in the form of exploitation or domination. This is a danger for healthcare given the vulnerability of patients, particularly patients from 'deprived' circumstances (Gilson, 2006). Also for groups living in poverty the consequences of misplaced trust can threaten livelihoods and lives (Coulson, 1998), and it may be easier to trust if you are powerful and wealthy. For some writers (Barbalet, 2005), trust works as a tranquiliser in social relations in which trust shuts down the trust giver's uncertainty in the face of the trust taker's freedom to act how they wish. Thus, given the potential benefits and cost of trusting, relationship research may need to explore what levels and forms of trust contribute to positive health outcomes and healthcare performance.

There appears, therefore, to be seemingly contradictory developments between the need to foster trust relationships at a number of different levels in the healthcare system and the demand for increased control over professionals and safety for the public (Kuhlmann, 2006). Certainly, there may be tension between the development of trust and other policy goals, in particular the development of patient empowerment. The notion of more active service users empowered to both actively manage their condition and participate in decision making regarding their treatment has been vigorously promoted for the positive benefits that such participation may produce. This may be contrasted with the more traditional patient role, which involved a passive approach and high, possibly blind trust in their clinician's decisions. If trust relations between patients and clinicians are becoming more conditional, can they still contribute positively to health outcomes? Patient empowerment is a key goal of the UK government's current approach to chronic disease management and it forms part of the changing context for trust relations in the NHS, to which we now turn.

The context – the case of the 'new NHS'

Public and patient trust in healthcare in the UK appears to be shaped by a variety of influences. From a macro perspective, any changes in levels of public trust in healthcare institutions appear to derive partly from top-down policy initiatives that have altered the way in which health services are organised and partly from changes in public attitudes to healthcare. The latter may be linked with how the NHS is run and financed and the pressure on NHS budgets due to increased demand by an ageing population, the rising costs of technology and increases in public sector pay (Taylor-Gooby and Hastie, 2003). Or it may be linked with broader social and cultural processes that are claimed to have produced a decline in deference to authority and trust in experts and institutions, increasing reliance on personal judgements of risk (Giddens, 1991; Beck, 1992; O'Neil, 2002), and which may be linked to an overall decline in social trust due to the breakdown of communities, social networks and cohesion (Putnam, 2000). Consumerist forces are proposed to have produced a shift in the balance of power within which trust relations are formed, changing public and professional vulnerabilities and the requirement for trust in their relationship (Newman, 1998). Institutional trust may have also been affected by negative media coverage of scandals over medical competence in the 1990s such as the inquiry into paediatric cardiac surgery in

Bristol, the conviction of the GP Harold Shipman and the removal of organs from children at Alder Hey hospital (Davies, 1999). Certainly, there is evidence to suggest that the public increasingly see the doctors' regulatory body, the General Medical Council, as self-interested even though public trust in doctors remains high (Allsop, 2006).

The change in public attitudes towards professionals and the emergence of more informed and potentially demanding patients that may have occurred as a result of these broader cultural processes provide a context for government policy that has positioned itself as seeking to make the NHS both more responsive to patients' needs and more efficient. Any change in interpersonal and institutional trust relations can be understood as the natural outcome of these wider changes in both government policy and social attitudes. In the next section we will examine how the UK government's policy initiative of clinical governance and the resulting use of performance management with heightened scrutiny of clinical activity may have affected both the professional discourse and forms of trust within the NHS.

Policy discourse – trust, clinical governance and performance management

The post-war consensus in the NHS in the UK, in which trust in professionalism underpinned the relationships between the public, health professions and the state (Newman, 1998), is believed to have been undermined by the growth of consumerism, by an erosion of the public service ethos due to the promotion of entrepreneurial values in the public sector (Brereton and Temple, 1999) and by political and media portrayals of professional activity as paternalistic. This high trust system of governance has been replaced by the gradual introduction of the new public management with its emphasis on regulation, audit and monitoring, which is believed to have brought with it a 'culture' of 'low trust' (Gilson, 2003; Rowe and Calnan, 2006) (see Figure 4.2). Since the Labour government came into power in 1997, performance management has been a central mechanism for reforming the way that services are delivered in the NHS. This target-driven approach has been applied to both managerial and clinical domains, with the introduction of assessment of clinical activity through the clinical governance initiative aimed at ensuring clinical accountability for the quality of care provided.

Increasing managerial monitoring of clinical activity has obvious consequences for trust relationships between providers and managers (Davies, 1999). Harrison and Smith (2004) argue that the new policy framework of clinical governance has sought to achieve a shift in focus from trust relationships between people to confidence in abstract systems, such as rules and regulations. The more behaviour is constrained by such systems, so uncertainty is reduced and visibility is increased (Giddens, 1990) and the less is the need to rely on trust (Smith, 2001). More recent Labour government policy in the UK has returned to the use of market mechanisms of governance to try to secure increased accountability and responsiveness of healthcare providers (see also Burau and Vrangbæk, this volume). Figure 4.2 illustrates how the type of governance approach can produce different levels of trust and suggests that neither new public management techniques nor market mechanisms will necessarily be effective in increasing public trust in the health service. It raises the question (Evetts, 2006) whether complex systems of accountability and control undermine trust and displace it with various criteria of performance and indicators for review and accounting or whether this new form of regulation encourages new strategies for building trust and challenges the powerful expert/lay divide in healthcare and the concept of professionalism itself (Kuhlmann, 2006).

Figure 4.2: The distribution of trust and state control in various models of governance

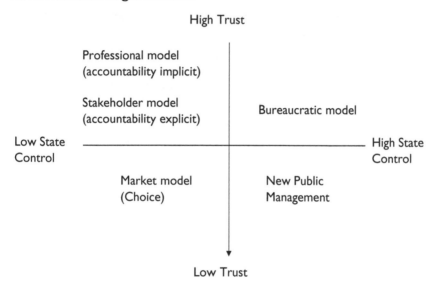

Empirical evidence to show whether credible external performance measurements build up confidence in organisations, requiring less trust in them, is not yet available. As Sheaff and colleagues (2004) noted in their scoping exercise for the Service Development Organisation (SDO), there has been limited empirical research evaluating the impact of external performance measures, particularly from the perspective of service users. Those studies that have explored this problem have reported quite negative findings. Mannion and Goddard's (2003) evaluation of the impact of the Clinical Resources and Audit Group (CRAG) clinical outcome indicators in Scotland reported limited use of such data by patients and GPs and also within hospital Trusts. Similarly, studies of the use of report cards in the US have found on the whole that published performance rarely stimulates quality improvement and the public distrusts and fails to make use of it. As Power (1997) argues, the growth of performance measurement and audit may merely result in 'certificates of comfort' offering reassurance that performance is being measured without resulting in change. Where trust is low, the reliability of the information published may be questioned and any uncertainty in the data and what it means may do little to increase public confidence in healthcare institutions.

The perverse incentives that may be generated by performance management systems, in that a system that 'does not trust people begets people that cannot be trusted' (Davies and Lampel, 1998, p 160), highlights the risk of gaming behaviour in such an approach. Obtaining a performance measure that is credible to providers, commissioners and service users and that enhances confidence in healthcare organisations is particularly pertinent when market mechanisms are being used to manage health service delivery.

Professional discourse and trust

This debate about the relative decline or not in trust in healthcare and in the institution of medicine should not be divorced from the wider discussion about the extent to which medical power and authority is on the wane, or that medicine, in the face of recent challenges, has managed to retain its overall dominance (Coburn et al, 1997). Sociological accounts (Freidson, 2001) of the professionalising strategies of medicine have consistently shown how, at least at the elite or macro level, medicine is able to respond to or anticipate possible challenges or changes and sometimes use the opportunities to maintain or even enhance its autonomy and control. One of the themes that runs through the current professional 'discourse' on trust is that the so-called decline in public trust – brought about by scandals such as Shipman – is a 'problem' for medicine that has led to the introduction of tighter mechanisms for regulation and accountability. It is difficult to know how far these changes were forced on the profession (Baker, 2004) or whether it, or certain sections of it, may have colluded with the state as it enhanced the project of modernising medicine. The modern medical professions' representatives appear to have associated themselves with the philosophy of the 'new professionalism', and central to this is a call to the public for a partnership based on mutual trust. The old concordat between the profession, the state and the public founded on self-regulation and paternalism would be replaced with a new one based on patient autonomy and patients' rights, greater accountability on the part of doctors and partnership (Irvine, 2003; DH, 2006, 2007; see also Allsop and Jones, and Burau and Vrangbæk, this volume).

This approach might be seen as another example of a professionalising strategy in that it is a way of fending off any further threats to autonomy by the state or through marketisation by emphasising the need for patients to trust doctors to self-regulate and to work together with them. In the past, professionalism and trust were presumed to be intrinsic to doctors' values and the doctor–patient relationship, whereas now professional bodies or their representatives feel the need to make them explicit. Similarly, it has been argued (Evetts, 2006) that there is an emergence or re-emergence of both an appeal to professionalism and trust in sociological theories of occupational control. Previous critical analysis of professionalism depicted occupations as driven primarily by self-interest and the need for power, status and material wealth. Trust was used as a means of duping the public into believing in the superior product of scientific medicine and thus enhancing the professionalising project. More recent theories have reconnected trust and professionalism through the renewed interest in risk and the challenges posed by a possible decline in public trust.

Other sociological accounts of the link between trust and professionalism (Kuhlmann, 2006) have shown how the medical profession have used the development of external regulation to reinforce their professional position. They suggest that the development of the new tools of bureaucratic regulation, which are signifiers of quality, are actively used by doctors to build trustful relations with colleagues. They are used as 'public proofs' of the quality of their services under conditions of tighter control and regulation. They are also taken up by patients and perceived as prerequisites for self-determined decisions and trustworthy relations. The traditional 'embodied' professionalism is transformed into a 'disembodied' professionalism founded on information. Thus, Kuhlmann (2006) argues that new patterns of building trust are emerging rather than being in decline. On this premise, exhortations by senior leaders within the medical profession for their colleagues to engage with and lead the implementation of 'clinical governance' may be interpreted as a further way for clinicians to protect their power base. Clinicians may be more explicitly accountable for the quality of care they provide, but they continue to define what quality is, how it is to be measured and how the results can be interpreted.

Theoretical framework for explaining trust relations in the 'new NHS'

A theoretical framework (see Table 4.1) can be drawn up based on the proposition that changes in the organisational structure of medical care and the culture of healthcare delivery have changed the experiences of healthcare for individual patients and affected trust relations between patients, providers and managers. These changes have in part been initiated by healthcare professionals, in part by the government, with clinical governance requirements that benchmark clinical performance and its policies on patient choice and the expert patient programme with its emphasis on shared decision making (Rowe and Calnan, 2006), and in part by patients or patient groups (Baggott et al, 2005), some of whom wish to be equal partners in treatment decisions. It is not proposed that these changes have cumulatively achieved a shift from trust in people to confidence in abstract systems. The provision of healthcare is still characterised by uncertainty and risk and there is evidence that not only are patients sceptical of institutional confidence-building mechanisms such as performance ratings, but that interactions between managers and clinicians continue to rely on informal relations and unwritten rules rather than performance management (Goddard and Mannion, 1998). Rather, it is proposed that new forms of trust relations are emerging in this new context of healthcare delivery, reflecting a change in motivations for trust from affective-based to cognition-based trust as patients, clinicians and managers are encouraged to become more active partners in trust relations.

It is proposed that provision of information and greater patient involvement in their care, through the attempted shift towards shared decision making in doctor–patient relationships, has produced greater interdependence between patients and clinicians. Certainly, in primary care, embodied trust (Green, 2004), arising out of an enduring relationship with the 'family doctor', may be less relevant, not least because of the structural changes that may have increased the range of points of access to primary healthcare and reduced the opportunities for continuity of care. For some patients, as their care may be provided by an increasing range of healthcare professionals, professional and educational credentials and status may no longer be sufficient guarantees that an individual clinician will provide the standard and type of care they want. It is possible that they may trust nurses or therapists to be competent in certain aspects of their care, but for other aspects may insist on seeing a doctor.

How can informed trust (see Table 4.1) be characterised from a patient's perspective and in what ways would it differ from a patient's perspectives on embodied trust? There are a number of possible dimensions. One is clearly in the area of decision making, where there would be an increasingly active patient involved in decision making who might expect doctors to trust their ability/competence to self-manage compared with the more passive and deferential role associated with paternalistic medicine. The second dimension involves the use of information. Informed trust might be associated with the use of information to calculate whether trust is warranted, whereas, with embodied trust, information may have been valued for the respect it shows rather than its content. In this way, patients may display a more rational rather than emotive response to information. Third, perspectives may differ on the willingness to take risks, in that informed trust may involve the patient carefully weighing up the situation, whereas embodied trust may involve the patient basing their judgement on the reputation of the organisation or individual. Finally, embodied trust implies that a clinician's altruism is unquestioned and the other party is well intentioned. This may be contrasted with informed trust where the patient may express greater suspicion and scepticism about others' intentions.

This shift towards informed, conditional trust may also depend on the patient's circumstances, needs and preferences and the context in which care is provided (Robb and Greenhalgh, 2006). For example, in Mechanic and Meyer's study (2000), patients with illnesses such as breast cancer were more likely to describe their trust relations as being unconditional than those with Lyme disease who had experienced difficulties in obtaining a diagnosis. Trust relations are also dynamic and may change during the pathway of care. For example, Thorne and Robinson (1989) reported that patients went from a naive, unconditional trust in diagnosis through to a more conditional, negotiated relationship as their treatment became more established. Similarly, the nature of trust relationships and the balance between affective-based and cognitive-based trust may vary according to the social position of the patient. The ability to adopt this more 'active' stance may depend on the extent to which patients have access to appropriate resources (such as finance, time and energy) (Gilson, 2003). It might also be argued that all trust relationships have a conditional element to them and that traditionally there has been widespread ambivalence about scientific medicine and medical practitioners (Calnan et al, 2005). The suggestion here is that conditionality has now become more explicit.

For GPs and hospital doctors, trust relations (see Table 4.1) may have changed between themselves and in their relations with other practitioners as the health service has emphasised the need to be primary care led and other healthcare professionals have become responsible for delivery of services, creating new relations in which trust has to be earned through collaboration rather than relying on peer trust. Thus, 'earned' trust might be characterised by an individual clinician's authority and reputation being based on their proven skills and competence, and being up to date with medical technology; trust gained by following agreed team-based protocols, imposing some limits to clinical freedom; successful relations between clinicians based on mutual respect for their different competencies and knowledge; and communication skills and providing information in building trust. This stands in marked contrast to more traditional relations of 'peer trust' where an individual clinician's authority and reputation are based on their position in the medical hierarchy, personal networks and word-of-mouth recommendation. Here hierarchical relations dominate, as clinical freedom is unquestioned, as are senior clinicians' views and decisions, performance is self-regulated, and successful relations between clinicians are based on conforming to traditional roles. Trust may be generally higher between clinicians of the same profession and specialty.

Finally, what of the changes in trust relations between managers and practitioners created primarily by the UK government's clinical governance policy? We argue that this has led to a change from a relationship characterised by status to one characterised by 'performance' (see Table 4.1). The former might be depicted as a one-way relationship with clinicians having little need to trust managers, whereas managers have to trust clinicians. A clinician's authority relates to their position and role within the organisation and managers act as administrators, trusting strategic decisions as to how services are to be delivered and how resources are to be used by clinicians. There would be minimal monitoring of activity and managers would not be involved in such assessments. In contrast, performance trust might involve a two-way relationship as clinicians need to work with managers to secure resources and to develop services, and managers have to work with clinicians to achieve their performance goals and to meet government targets. A clinician's authority would be related to their involvement in managerial activity and their ability to meet targets, as well as their position within the organisation and clinical skills. Trust would be important in successful clinician–manager relations as it reduces the need for monitoring and may produce greater job satisfaction, higher staff retention and more efficient organisational performance.

Table 4.1: Conceptual framework for explaining trust relations in the new NHS

Relationship	Trustor		Trustee		Context	Type of trust
	Affect based	Cognition based	Reputation based on status	Reputation based on performance		
Traditional clinician–patient	X		X		Paternalistic medicine	Embodied trust
Traditional clinician–clinician		X	X		Autonomous self-regulation/hierarchical	Peer trust
Traditional clinician–manager	X		X		Professional autonomy/expertise	Status trust
New NHS clinician–patient	X	X	X	X	Expert patient	Informed trust
New NHS clinician–clinician		X		X	Shared care	Earned trust
New NHS clinician–manager		X		X	Clinical governance	Performance trust

This general typology of trust relations outlined in the framework (see Table 4.1) suggests that trust relations in all three types of relationship in the 'new' modernised NHS might, in general, be characterised by an emphasis on communication, providing information and the use of 'evidence' to support decisions in a reciprocal, negotiated alliance.

The question remains about how trust relations in healthcare compare with those in other sections of welfare and public sector services. Have the 'unique' characteristics of the healthcare setting proved more resistant to organisational and social changes that may have eroded or changed trust relations in other settings, or is 'conditional trust' now common in service provision throughout the public sector? There is also the question of whether trust is still as politically salient now as it was in the late 1990s. The 1997 UK Labour administration had a distinctly 'communitarian turn' with its emphasis on the rights and responsibilities of citizens and citizen engagement in institutional governance, and the importance of inter- and intra-agency cooperation in the production of social capital. In contrast, the current direction of government policy with its emphasis on individual choice and the marketisation of public services may have a cumulative negative impact on social capital.

As government policy increasingly seeks to introduce contestability into the NHS, it raises new questions as to the role and optimal level of trust in commissioning services from a variety of providers. This new policy context is likely to change the nature of vulnerabilities and risks to which patients, clinicians and managers are exposed, which in turn will affect both the relevance and nature of trust in healthcare relationships.

References

Alaszweski, A. (2003) 'Risk, trust and health', Editorial, *Health, Risk and Society*, vol 5, no 3, pp 235-40.

Allsop, J. (2006) 'Regaining trust in medicine: professional and state strategies', *Current Sociology*, vol 54, no 4, pp 621-36.

Anheier, H.K. and Kendall, J. (2002) 'Interpersonal trust and voluntary associations', *British Journal of Sociology*, vol 53, no 3, pp 343-60.

Baggott, R., Allsop, J. and Jones, K. (2005) *Speaking for patients and carers*, Basingstoke: Palgrave.

Baker, R. (2004) 'Patient-centred care after Shipman', *Journal of the Royal Society of Medicine*, vol 97, no 4, pp 161-5.

Barbalet, J. (2005) 'Trust and uncertainty: the emotional basis of rationality', ESRC meeting, London School of Economics and Political Science, December.

Barber, B. (1983) *The logic and limits of trust*, New Brunswick, NJ: Rutgers University Press.

Beck, U. (1992) *Risk society*, London: Sage Publications.

Brereton, M. and Temple, M. (1999) 'The new public service ethos: an ethical environment for governance', *Public Administration*, vol 77, no 3, pp 455-74.

Calnan, M. and Rowe, R. (2004) *Trust in health care: An agenda for future research*, London: The Nuffield Trust.

Calnan, M. and Rowe, D. (2006) 'Researching trust relations in health care: conceptual and methodological challenges', *Journal of Health Organization and Management*, vol 20, no 5, pp 349-58.

Calnan, M., Montaner, D. and Horne, R. (2005) 'How acceptable are innovative health care technologies? A survey of public beliefs and attitudes in England and Wales', *Social Science and Medicine*, vol 60, pp 1937-48.

Coburn, R., Rappolt, S. and Bourgeault, I.L. (1997) 'Decline vs retention of medical power through restratification; the Ontario case', *Sociology of Health and Illness*, vol 19, no 1, pp 1-22.

Coulson, A. (1998) 'Trust and contract in public sector management', in A. Coulson (ed) *Trust and contracts: Relationships in local government health and public services*, Bristol: The Policy Press, pp 9-34.

Davies, H. (1999) 'Falling public trust in health services: implications for accountability', *Journal of Health Services Research Policy*, vol 4, no 4, pp 193-4.

Davies, H. and Lampel, J. (1998) 'Trust in performance indicators', *Quality in Health Care*, vol 7, pp 159-62.

DH (Department of Health) (2006) *Good doctors, safer patients*, London: The Stationery Office.

DH (2007) *Trust assurance and safety – the regulation of health professionals in the 21st century*, London: The Stationery Office.

Evetts, J. (2006) 'Introduction, trust and professionalism: challenges and occupational changes', *Current Sociology*, vol 54, no 4, pp 607-20.

Freidson, E. (2001) *Professionalism: The third logic*, Cambridge: Polity Press.

Gambetta, D. (1998) *Trust: Making and breaking cooperative relations*, Oxford: Blackwell.

Giddens, A. (1990) *The consequences of modernity*, Cambridge: Polity Press.

Giddens, A. (1991) *Modernity and self-identity: Self and society in the late modern age*, Cambridge: Polity Press.

Gilson, L. (2003) 'Trust and the development of health care as a social institution', *Social Science and Medicine*, vol 56, pp 1453-68.

Gilson, L. (2006) 'Trust and health care: theoretical perspectives and research needs', *Journal of Health Organization and Management*, vol 20, pp 359-75.

Gilson, L., Palmer, N. and Schneider, H. (2005) 'Trust and health worker performance: exploring a conceptual framework using South African evidence', *Social Science and Medicine*, vol 61, pp 1418-29.

Goddard, M. and Mannion, R. (1998) 'From competition to co-operation: new economic relationships in the National Health Service', *Health Economics*, vol 7, pp 105-19.

Green, J. (2004) 'Is trust an under-researched component of healthcare organisation?', *British Medical Journal*, vol 329, p 384.

Hall, M., Dogan, E., Zheng, B. and Mishra, A. (2001) 'Trust in physicians and medical institutions: does it matter?', *The Milbank Quarterly*, vol 79, pp 613-39.

Harrison, S. and Smith, C. (2004) 'Trust and moral motivation: redundant resources in health and social care?', *Policy & Politics*, vol 32, pp 371-86.

Irvine, D. (2003) *The doctor's tale: Professionalism and the public trust*, Oxford: Radcliffe Medical Press.

Kuhlmann, E. (2006) 'Traces of doubt and sources of trust: health professions in an uncertain society', *Current Sociology*, vol 54, no 4, pp 607-20.

Lewicki, R. and Bunker, B. (1996) 'Developing and maintaining trust in work relationships', in R. Kramer and R. Tyler (eds) *Trust in organizations: Frontiers of theory and research*, Thousand Oaks, CA: Sage Publications, pp 114-39.

Luhmann, N. (1979) *Trust and power*, Chichester: Wiley.

Mannion, R. and Goddard, M. (2003) 'Public disclosure of comparative clinical performance data: lessons from the Scottish experience', *Journal of Evaluation of Clinical Practice*, vol 9, pp 2277-86.

Mayer, R., Davis, J. and Schoorman, F. (1995) 'An integrative model of organization trust', *Academic Management Review*, vol 23, pp 438-58.

Mechanic, D. (1998) 'Functions and limits of trust in providing medical care', *Journal of Health Politics, Policy and Law*, vol 23, pp 661-86.

Mechanic, D. and Meyer, S. (2000) 'Concepts of trust among patients with serious illness', *Social Science and Medicine*, vol 51, pp 657-68.

Mishra, A. (1996) 'Organizational responses to crisis: the centrality of trust', in R. Kramer and T. Tyler (eds) *Trust in organizations: Frontiers of theory and research*, Thousand Oaks, CA: Sage Publications, pp 261-87.

Newman, J. (1998) 'The dynamics of trust', in A. Coulson (ed) *Trust and contracts: Relationships in local government, health and public services*, Bristol: The Policy Press, pp 35-51.

O'Neil, O. (2002) *A question of trust, BBC Reith lectures*, Cambridge: Cambridge University Press.

Power, M. (1997) *The audit society: Rituals of verification*, Oxford: Oxford University Press.

Putnam, R. (2000) *Bowling alone: The collapse and revival of American community*, New York: Simon and Schuster.

Robb, N. and Greenhalgh, T. (2006) 'You have to cover up the words of the doctor: the mediation of trust in interpreted consultations in primary care', *Health Organization and Management*, vol 20, pp 434-55.

Rose-Ackerman, S. (2001) 'Trust, honesty and corruption: reflection on the state-building process', *European Journal of Sociology*, vol 42, pp 526-70.

Rowe, R. and Calnan, M. (2006) 'Trust relations in health care: developing a theoretical framework for the "new" NHS', *Journal of Health Organization and Management*, vol 20, pp 376-96.

Safran, D., Taira, D., Rogers, W., Kosinski, M., Ware, J. and Tarlov, A. (1998) 'Linking primary care performance to outcomes of care', *Journal of Family Practice*, vol 47, no 3, pp 213-20.

Sheaff, R., Mashall, M., Rogers, A., Roland, M., Sibbald, B. and Pickard, S. (2004) 'Governmentality by network in English primary healthcare', *Social Policy & Administration*, vol 38, no 1, pp 89-103.

Smith, C. (2001) 'Trust and confidence: possibilities for social work in "high modernity"', *British Journal of Social Work*, vol 31, pp 287-305.

Taylor-Gooby, P. and Hastie, C. (2003) 'Paying for world class services: a British dilemma', *Journal of Social Policy*, vol 32, pp 271-88.

Thom, D. and Ribisi, K. (1999) 'Further validation and reliability testing of the trust in physician scale', *Medical Care*, vol 37, pp 510-17.

Thom, D., Hall, M. and Pawlson, L. (2004) 'Measuring patients' trust in their physicians when assessing quality of care', *Health Affairs*, vol 23, no 4, pp 124-32.

Thorne, D. and Robinson, C.A. (1989) 'Guarded alliance: health care relationships in chronic illness', *Journal of Nursing Scholarship*, vol 21, pp 3153-7.

Titmuss, R. (1968) *Commitment to welfare*, London: Allen and Unwin.

Tyler, R. and Kramer, R. (1996) 'Whither trust?', in R. Kramer and T. Tyler (eds) *Trust in organizations: Frontiers of theory and research*, Thousand Oaks, CA: Sage Publications, pp 1-15.

Warren, M.E. (1999) *Democracy and trust*, Cambridge: Cambridge University Press.

FIVE

Professionalism meets entrepreneurialism and managerialism[1]

Rosalie A. Boyce

Introduction

The shift in recent decades towards free-market economics, competition and 'small government' policies in Western liberal democracies has led to an ideological and political climate that has favoured a suite of reformist activity characterised in the literature as 'new public management' (Pollitt, 1990). New public management (NPM) is not simply a set of new management practices but a form of deep restructuring drawing together the principles of managerialism and marketisation into context-specific priorities for change in the public sector. Underpinning reform directions is the belief in the superiority of private sector management principles, organisational forms and market-based mechanisms in producing value for public money, greater public choice, increased efficiency and increased responsiveness to customers (Hood, 1991, 1995).

Hood (1995) has shown that the policy mix and intensity of NPM reform varies according to national context. Thus, although there are similar general approaches or policy instruments discernable across national contexts, specific outcomes depend on the underlying geopolitical arrangements. Although some countries have pulled back from the implementation of the more radical aspects of NPM policies, we note that at the institutional level of health service agencies the pressures on public sector professionals to pursue competitive and enterprising modes of conduct, and the operational processes that condition them, have persisted. This state of active commercial focus at the institutional level has resulted in part from contests over a diminishing resource base (Flynn, 1998) and from the direct appeals to health professionals for more 'business-like' practices.

The purpose of this chapter is to examine the implication of NPM-styled reforms on professional culture and practices in public sector health services using the Australian allied health professions as the case study. The particular focus is on the repertoire of conducts that professionals mobilise in the face of challenges posed by NPM-styled reforms. The chapter addresses this aim by first discussing the impact of NPM-styled reforms on the professions generally before turning the focus to public sector health professions and entrepreneurship specifically. The research context and methodology are then introduced, including an explanation of the research subjects – allied health professions – before the findings are examined.

Health sector reform, the professions and enterprise discourse

A general theme in the NPM literature is the challenge that NPM approaches such as marketisation and managerialism mount to traditional professional practices and interests. The challenge to professional power reflects the market liberalist abhorrence of anti-competitive monopolies that restrict consumer choice and enhance producer power (Exworthy and Halford, 1998). Typical NPM-styled approaches to circumventing professional power have found expression in reforms related to the elimination of anti-competitive barriers, greater accountability, transparent and quantifiable performance management systems, and quasi-markets to garner greater responsiveness to consumers. A key conclusion from the corpus of literature is that the professions and the organisations they inhabit are in transition in a complex and interacting process of responding and adapting to and resisting and in some cases appropriating aspects of the reform agenda (Exworthy and Halford, 1998).

Understanding many of the drivers affecting contemporary professional practices in this reform environment is assisted by a consideration of the discourse of enterprise and its role in conditioning change. Although critical debates have emerged as to the role of enterprise culture in terms of overgeneralised and deterministic accounts of its hegemonic status (Fournier and Grey, 1999), there is support for the claim that as a rhetorical device it has served 'a prime function as a justificatory discourse for massive changes' in the restructuring of national public sectors (Burrows, 1991, p 10). Hence, enterprise discourse looms large in the research context of this chapter, specifically in terms of the cajoling discourse for professionals to be more enterprising, business-like and customer-focused.

The strain between professional and enterprise discourses has been captured by Fournier (2000). Her analysis noted the tension between the celebratory fervour for flexibility and 'boundarylessness' inherent in the discourse of NPM and enterprise and the importance of boundaries for the professions (see also Wrede, this volume). Within such apparent contradictory tensions lie further grounds for the reconstructing and renegotiating of professions and their identity and practices (see also Dahle and Skogheim, this volume). Following on from Fournier's (1999) approach of disciplinary logic, and the Foucauldian notion of governmentality (Foucault, 1991), the deployment of appeals to the discursive resources of enterprise culture serves as a disciplining logic in attempts to condition a new-fashioned professionalism. It is at the juncture where professional culture meets enterprise culture in the institutional-level context of a raft of NPM-styled reforms and constrained resources that this chapter is situated.

A small body of work has been published on entrepreneurial activity in the health professions (Ennew et al, 1998a, 1998b; Calnan et al, 2000; Richardson and Cullen, 2000; Powell and Barnett, 2001). A theme in these works is that the role of resource allocator and coordinator was fundamental to the nature of the public sector entrepreneur. Entrepreneurial activity was characterised as the willingness to exploit the added flexibility, efficiency and discretion arising from opportunities for change. There was also evidence of entrepreneurial orientation and business-like activities, but resistance to self-identifying as an entrepreneur. The studies of Ennew and colleagues (1998a, 1998b) and Powell and Barnett (2001) rely on a notion of entrepreneurialism based on the formation of new models of organisation. This approach is consistent with Thornton's (1999) review of the sociology of entrepreneurship that defines entrepreneurship as 'the creation of new organizations [...] which occurs as a context-dependent, social and economic process' (p 20). Entrepreneurial activity is conceptualised as a form of public utility for the benefit of patient services rather than for personal profit. For the purposes of this chapter we follow the general approach of the works cited above in terms of the conceptualisation of public sector entrepreneurialism.

The empirical studies conducted to date have concentrated on medical and dental settings. How then do other professions that make up the much-vaunted multidisciplinary healthcare team respond to the same appeals for more business-like modes of organisation and practice? How do they exercise their role and what is their attitude to such changes in terms of the forces being brought to bear on established forms of professional conduct? These questions are addressed in this study of Australian allied health professions working in public sector general hospitals. In the following section, key features of the research context and methodology are presented. We begin with a brief description of the allied health professions and sketch the state of organisational change in the Australian health sector.

The allied health professions

In the Australian context up to 19 professional disciplines are accepted as allied health professions ranging from the better-known disciplines of physiotherapy, occupational therapy, speech pathology, psychology, pharmacy and dietetics to the less well-known podiatry and orthodics (Boyce, 2004). The closest similar context is that of the UK and the 'professions supplementary to medicine' (also referred to as the 'professions allied to medicine') where 12 professions are recognised as part of the cluster and numbers are on the increase (Larkin, 2002). Historically informed Anglo-American studies of the development of the allied health professions have concluded that they have been subject to medical dominance through limitations on their autonomy (Willis, 1989; Øvretveit, 1992; Larkin, 2002). Within these overarching constraints, allied health professionals enjoy significant levels of autonomy, particularly at the technical level of decision making about the services clients are to receive, and at the practice level of authority over the organisation of their work (Øvretveit, 1992; Boyce, 1997).

Professional authority over the organisation of their work is apparent from the longstanding tradition in Australia and Anglo–American countries of professional hierarchies under profession-based management. The rise of managerialism and marketisation strategies in the health sector from the late 1980s in the UK and the early 1990s in Australia disrupted the stable order of professional hierarchies and provided opportunities for new roles, new managerial and budgetary responsibilities and new organisational forms (Øvretveit, 1992; Mays and Pope, 1997; Borthwick, 2000). For example, Øvretveit's (1992) British study found evidence of 'business autonomy' arising from the accrual of contract-based service revenue flows. Table 5.1 summarises key features of the impact of NPM-styled reforms on the Australian allied health professions.

Organisational change in the Australian health sector

Public hospitals in Australia are the responsibility of the eight state and territory governments, not the federal government. As a result, there is a complex geopolitical landscape. Hood (1991) observed that in Australia a 'business-type managerialism' was the more prominent of NPM-styled reforms. Although there was never any full-blown separation of purchasers and providers in a quasi-market arrangement similar to that in the UK or New Zealand, the mid-1990s did witness an increased use of marketisation and competition-based strategies such as compulsory competitive tendering programmes, privatisation strategies, service contestability and private finance partnership initiatives across a range of sectors. Health professions undertook a range of preparatory performance benchmarking and costing exercises. Despite a subsequent general pullback of support by the states and territories for market testing clinical services, these anticipatory preparations were normalised into the organisational routines of many allied health professions because of institutional-level pressures from hospital managers for more business-like and evidence-based practice (Boyce, 2004).

Governance of Australian hospitals has changed markedly since the early 1990s. The traditional triumvirate approach has been largely restructured into decentralised, financially accountable, medically managed clinical units (Braithwaite and Westbrook, 2005). Table 5.2 describes some of the key features of restructured Australian public hospitals compared to the pre-reform era. The Australian decentralised clinical units and clinician manager roles are quite similar to the British-styled clinical directorate (Kitchener, 2000) with one important exception that is central to the current study. In Australia the allied health professions were almost without exception not incorporated within the clinical unit model. The dominant new organisational model for Australian allied health professions in public hospitals by 2000 was to stand outside the medically managed clinical units in their own divisional structure under the leadership and management of a new non-medical and non-nursing leadership position: the

Table 5.1: Comparison of Australian allied health professions in the public hospital sector, pre- and post-NPM-styled reform

Dimensions	Pre-NPM-styled reform, until 1990	Post-NPM-styled reform, 1990 onwards
Financial	Historical allocated budgets administered by profession manager through the medical director	Institutional-level internal purchaser–provider models become widespread based on service agreements; some examples of zero-based budgeting
Institutional policy environment	Promotes active stewardship of budget through cost containment	Promotes expectations of building revenue base through external contracts or grants
Organisational model	Individual profession hierarchies within a medical division; individual profession managers report to a medical director	Profession hierarchies gather under the collective of an allied health division; individual profession managers report to a director of allied health
Executive-level representation	Subsumed within medical representative structure	First examples of self-representation occur through a director or chairperson of allied health
Professional autonomy (contingent)	Technical/clinical; practice organisation level	Technical/clinical; practice organisation level; institutional-level autonomy through self-representation; business autonomy
Professional identity	Internal focus on the professional discipline identity, for instance physiotherapy	Interprofessional focus on building a collective allied health subculture at an institutional level while maintaining the discipline identities at the clinical level

director of allied health (Boyce, 2001). The formation of allied health divisions as managerial business units theoretically set up a framework for an internal purchaser–provider/purchaser–supplier relationship with medically managed clinical units/directorates, with the attendant possibility of increased 'business autonomy'.

The primary focus of the research to be reported here was to examine the impact of appeals for more enterprising and business-like conduct on public sector allied health professionals. The uptake of internal service agreements, external contracting of services to third parties and restructuring into new forms

Table 5.2: Key features of restructured Australian public hospitals, pre- and post-NPM-styled reform

Features	Pre-NPM-styled reform, until 1990	Post-NPM-styled reform, 1990 onwards
Policy environment	Hospitals not directly managed by state health departments but subject to close relationship in terms of operational guidance; no policy support for a full-blown purchaser–provider model but recognition that new policy tools are needed to arrest growing public outlays on health services	Greater separation of the role of the state as funder and hospitals as operational providers; hospitals have greater autonomy in terms of ability to manage independently but intensity of performance management reporting framework increases; some services subjected to compulsory competitive tendering
Organisational structure	Hospitals are typically standalone entities with centralised decision-making structures	Widespread emergence of regional, district and area health board models; greater decentralisation with operational units accepting increased accountability for resource utilisation
Key governance approach	Triumvirate structure involving nursing, medicine and administration hierarchies	Clinical units are core business units of the organisation; medical, nursing and support staff decentralised to units
Financial	Historical allocated budgets; professional hierarchies act as internal budget holders expending their allocated resources; funded fully by public money	Output-based funding models, for example, case-mix funding, population-based funding; decentralised clinical units more prominent as accountable budget holders; public–private finance initiatives, for instance, co-locations
Professional staff	Exclusive focus on professional/clinical issues	Routine involvement in operational, financial and strategic decision making

of organisation were operationalised as indicators of a shift to an NPM-styled environment. These operational approaches represent significant and challenging departures from longstanding professional practices in public sector health services. In order to address the research questions a qualitative, inductive, multi-methods approach involving four longitudinal case studies was undertaken. The outcomes of NPM-styled reforms are best studied through detailed micro-level case studies that make visible the activity of actors and the specific organisational milieu conditioned by new management practices (Richardson and Cullen, 2000).

Case study sites were identified following the analysis of a national telephone survey of all Australian general hospitals with more than 100 beds (N=107 hospitals, 94% participation rate). The survey established the extent of operational indicators of NPM-styled reforms referred to above. The research design purposefully targeted high experience sites for the case studies because the phenomenon was accessible in a more stable form than would be available at other less experienced sites. Two phases of data collection were conducted between 1999 and 2001. It was an agreement under ethical approval that the identity of the case studies not be revealed and quotations from the study be notated in an anonymous style that protects the identity of interviewees.

A criticism of studies about professionals facing managerialist and marketisation reforms is the failure to adequately specify the nature of the engagement with managerial roles (Causer and Exworthy, 1998). It is important to note that the allied health department head – not the divisional director – in Australian hospitals is a longstanding formal managerial role. The position of director of allied health – the divisional director role – emerged contemporaneously with the new position of medical clinician managers leading clinical units/directorates in the late 1980s. However, unlike the medical clinician manager, the allied health director incumbents are not neophyte managers as they are typically drawn from the ranks of experienced departmental managers leading profession-based hierarchies. The following sections of the chapter present the results of the study organised around three analytical themes relating to the modes of conduct associated with entrepreneurial professionalism: strategic entrepreneurs, calculative entrepreneurs and reluctant entrepreneurs.

Entrepreneurial modes of conduct

The primary data source is the narrative accounts of the allied health professionals from four case study sites, drawing on the different discourses they used to make sense of new modes of conduct and the implications for established forms of professionalism. Following Du Gay (1993) and Thornton (1999) these types of entrepreneurial action are not seen as part of a trait-based theory of personality or individual attributes. Rather, they are structured as 'modes of conduct' that involve the allocation of 'particular capacities and predispositions to individuals which enable them to become certain sorts of person' (Du Gay, 1993, p 645).

Strategic entrepreneurs

A small cohort of strategic entrepreneurs engaged in a purposeful, externally focused and ambitious programme of organisational and professional change was identified from the case studies. The focus of their activities was to extend the influence and resource base of allied health spanning the dual domains of the local workplace and the wider policy environment. For strategic entrepreneurs it was not simply a question of reconciling or balancing the competing interests of the professions and managerialism. Rather it was a case of using the reformist agenda to further the professional project through refashioning traditional concepts of professionalism. A question about what allied health professionals needed to do to be successful in the reform environment brought this response:

> 'I think they need to change their definition of professionalism ... they need to understand that they're not going to be able to effectively compete for scarce resources and provide the services down the track unless they become good at other things than besides treating [names a clinical condition]. So I think, if you want it in essence, they have to change the way they perceive professionalism and professional practice.' (#1-4-1)

A key part of the 'new' professionalism was to build collective strength through downplaying, but not rejecting, the separatist agenda of the individual allied health disciplines in favour of adopting an overarching professional identity that was consistent with the focus on the nation – allied health – rather than the tribe constituted by individual disciplines (Boyce, 2006a). Strategic entrepreneurs exhibited a conscious awareness of the attractiveness of engaging with managerialism and marketisation (Moran, 1998). Strategic entrepreneurs clearly saw their interests being furthered by being able to talk 'management' and master the technologies of managerialism.

Strategic entrepreneurs engaged in modes of conduct that exemplified the competitive culture of the private sector where risk taking was expected, an enterprising orientation was valued and external contracts were vigorously pursued. For example, the case study site characterised as reflecting the highest level of strategic entrepreneurial modes of conduct used the metaphor of the enterprising corporation to describe their model of collective self-management (Rowe et al, 2004). The division of allied health was viewed as a corporation or firm based on a boardroom model in which the director of allied health held the role of chairperson of the board and the managing professionals were shareholders – not stakeholders. Underpinning this approach to entrepreneurial governance is the articulation of the 'new' professionalism that was dependent on a commitment to collective identity and action:

'We run on a boardroom, that's how we run our senior stuff ... as the chairman of the board, I have responsibility to the board to meet their needs, so do the senior professional staff. So we use that boardroom mentality and then everyone in allied health is a shareholder, so therefore they have a responsibility to improve the company's profitability and public image. I know it's a bit of a game but it's about reframing something into a metaphor that people can understand, so therefore you can't go bagging allied health, because you're a shareholder. And as a shareholder you have a voice and you have a voting right and therefore you must keep your company's profits, what ever it is.' (#1-4-1)

Strategic entrepreneurs have a national vision and devote their energies to focusing on future positioning to embrace opportunities and to shape the emergence of opportunities. Their ambitious attempts at system-level change included strategies such as lobbying the political and policy apparatus of the state about the 'new' allied health and evangelical messages promoting a change agenda for the professions:

'I spend my life, as you know, travelling around Australia talking to people about how to promote allied health, how to do outcomes, how to plan, how to be an advocate about the market, about service agreements, about clinical costing, about um all of those things, and I've been doing it for a long time.' (#1-4-1)

Calculative entrepreneurs

A key difference between strategic entrepreneurs and calculative entrepreneurs is the focus of their vision, the reach of their influence objectives, their attitudes to risk and the more conservative nature of their strategies. Calculative entrepreneurs have a more modest ambition, focusing on the operational environment of their organisational context. They have a more cautious engagement with risk taking. They prefer to focus on innovations in internal costing and information technologies and the needs of internal purchasers in preference to pursuing high-profile, and sometimes high-risk, external revenue generation. Compared to strategic entrepreneurs, calculative entrepreneurs are less concerned about influencing policy and pursuing a national agenda to develop the 'new' professionalism in allied health, although they do contribute to such debates. Interview questions to calculative entrepreneurs about what allied health professionals need to do to be successful in the reform environment would elicit replies about data and outcome measurement, internal organisational arrangements or specific management skills:

'I think they have to be quite objective about what they do and what they really change.... They need to be able to see evidence-based practice and outcome measures as vital to their day-to-day functioning. Rather than just seeing it as an extra on top of what they do with their clinical work. So they need to actually have that imbedded in what they actually do.' (#2-5-1)

Calculative entrepreneurs, in common with strategic entrepreneurs, shared this investment in data systems long before the arrival of NPM-styled reforms dictated their development. However, while strategic entrepreneurs would take risks and innovate in a situation of imperfect information, seeing it as a first-mover strategy, calculative entrepreneurs were less stimulated by such risks until they had adequate data. In keeping with their more modest ambitions, calculative entrepreneurs had a more local view of achieving influence based on placing representatives on all organisational decision-making bodies and aligning themselves with players perceived as powerful. This organisational strategy is infused with the 'new' professionalism ordered around the collective identity of allied health rather than the traditional separatist agenda of individual professions:

'I think we need to align ourselves with some of the power players in the hospitals… And I think by becoming allied health divisions … now that we've reorganised ourselves into clusters and teams, there is much more of a presence. An allied health presence rather than individual departments and working closely, well the aim is to work more closely with the divisions, patients care units in the hospital. I think those things are all very positive.' (#3-3-1)

Reluctant entrepreneurs

The category of reluctant entrepreneurs reflects a cautious ambivalence and uncertainty about whether the effort of engaging with reform in their specific organisational context would result in better outcomes for the health professions and their clients. Evidence of reluctant entrepreneurs in the cohort was limited to small numbers. A hallmark was their distinct preference for operating in the relative safety of the clinical environment. Reluctant entrepreneurs typically explain the decision not to engage with NPM reforms as 'we looked at it but it was too much work', considering that already limited resources from the clinical care domain would need to be diverted towards the management domain of system design and implementation.

Reluctant entrepreneurs did not perceive themselves as risk averse. Rather they perceived that they were concentrating on their core business of clinical care, an environment in which they felt relatively secure compared to the demands of proactively engaging with managerialist-styled changes. Some reluctant entrepreneurs espoused uncertainty about whether success in meeting managerialist objectives would in fact be rewarded:

> 'When we were told we had to form into a business unit... They were looking at us pursuing um, boosting our budgets with money that we earned externally. There was no guarantee that if we earned money that our budgets inside would stay the same. It was probably, earn money, cut your budget, earn money, cut your budget, so there was really ... not a great incentive.' (#2-1-1)

A director of allied health who fitted the profile of the calculative entrepreneur reflected on the growing reluctance of their allied health department heads in the second round of data collection at the site:

> 'But it's [entrepreneurship is] a double-edged sword because in fact the more opportunities you pursue to get money to do things, I think the clearer it is that the public money tends to disappear. So, and it actually takes an awful lot of effort and time to create those partnerships to get that money. So if I'm doing all of that, or doing it with my heads of departments, then it's an opportunity cost. So instead of getting on with what we think we're supposed to be getting on with, core business, we're actually getting on with entrepreneurship.' (#3-1-2)

Although some allied health professionals displayed ambivalence and uncertainty about the reform agenda, it did not resonate fully with the 'unwilling compliance' category in the study of education sector managing professionals (Gleeson and Shain, 1999) or with the 'disenchanted' British GPs in the study of Ennew and colleagues (1998a).

Entrepreneurial professionalism

The aim of this chapter was to examine the implications of NPM-styled reforms on professional culture and practices in public sector health services. A key finding from the research is that professionalism is being subjected to reforming pressures that contribute to a shift towards 'entrepreneurial professionalism' in which the possession of managerialist and entrepreneurial skills is increasingly valued by the professionals themselves. Although a range of responses from professionals is evident in the study cohort, all were aware of the demands for, and possibilities of, repositioning professional practices around a more business-like focus. This emergent entrepreneurial dimension of a professional culture was expressed through different modes of conduct: strategic, calculative and reluctant.

Entrepreneurial professionalism was sustained by the justificatory discourse of enterprise and appeals for health professionals to display business-like behaviours. However, it was not simply a case of enterprise culture or the 'spreading logic of the market' (Fournier, 2000) overwhelming traditional professional culture. On the contrary, entrepreneurial professionalism, at least as practised by the study cohort of strategic entrepreneurs and calculative entrepreneurs, involved mastering the 'accounting' and 'accountability' inherent in these 'micro-technologies of management' (Dent, 2003) that were perceived as potentially harmful to professional interests (Aldridge, 1996).

While the medical profession might eschew costing and performance-based managerial instruments as a threat to their autonomy (Harrison and Dowswell, 2002), some segments of the allied health professions perceive that these approaches can be helpful to allied health's professionalising aspirations at the institutional and health system level. By displaying faultless performativity (Dent and Whitehead, 2002) and entrepreneurial vision these actors were able to make visible their professional and organisational contribution, a contribution that was traditionally obscured by the nature of their relationship with the dominant profession of medicine in the pre-reform environment (Boyce, 2006b).

Entrepreneurial professionals act as agents of NPM embracing the philosophy and practices of marketisation and managerialism; however, they are not exclusively in its service. The strategic entrepreneurs in particular exhibited a conscious recognition of the 'fit' between their long-term pre-reform objectives for a refashioning of traditional allied health professionalism and the 'opportunity structures' presented from the NPM implementation framework. As noted by Fournier (2000) the spreading logic of the market plays a role in the legitimation of (NPM-styled) strategies that professionals can use to maintain and progress the professional project.

Our analysis suggests a coupling and interconnection between 'old-' and 'new-' fashioned professionalism such that values and practices from each can be articulated within a framework of entrepreneurial professionalism. Entrepreneurial professionalism is a refashioning of traditional professionalism, not a rejection of it. For example, commitment to traditional professional values was evident through the desire to use 'business autonomy' revenues to cross-subsidise professional development activities and less well-resourced areas of public sector clinical practice. Entrepreneurial professionalism was enacted through three primary strategies in the case study sites: first, through developing a new collective culture of allied health; second, through the formation of new structural and leadership arrangements within health service agencies to propagate the culture; and, third, through the growth in institutionally and professionally valued business autonomy, which arose from pursuing internal service agreements and external contracts (Øvretveit, 1992; Boyce, 2006a).

The current study offers some original insights into the nature of entrepreneurial professionalism that differ from prior studies on the health professions. Specifically, in relation to the Australian allied health professions, entrepreneurialism can be understood in terms of attempts to develop a collective culture and identity at the workplace level and at the health system level (Boyce, 2006a). Collectivity and the remaking of professional identity and relationships created the platform for a range of 'profitable' new business endeavours that delivered independence and influence through revenues associated with business autonomy.

The development of an allied health culture required the allied health disciplines to 'buy in' to an approach, which would build new 'lateral solidarities' (Exworthy and Halford, 1998) across discipline boundaries. This strategy involved a realignment of traditional boundaries that have underpinned much of the history of these professions. Tribalism had to be overcome in order to construct an identity of allied health based on a new high-trust self-managing model independent of medicine and its traditional role of adjudicating turf wars between the disciplines (Boyce, 1997; Rowe et al, 2004). The goal of entrepreneurial allied health professionals was to reposition themselves in the medically dominated hierarchy of the workplace, and especially for strategic entrepreneurs, to reposition the allied health professions in the healthcare division of labour more generally at the level of the health system. This was accomplished through refashioning the traditional notion of allied health as allied to medicine towards a self-constituted identity anchored in the notion of allied health as allied to each other. This finding is significant, as prior research has typically remarked on the breakdown of 'lateral solidarities' within professional entities facing NPM-styled reforms rather than the building of new 'lateral solidarities'.

Structural reform, for example GP fundholding, was an important conditioning mechanism or 'opportunity structure' in the research context of the studies reviewed above on entrepreneurship in the health professions. Whittington and colleagues (1994, p 843) in their study of market-driven change in professional services in particular noted that 'decentralization offers professionals new areas of opportunity and discretion, new ways of playing political games or exercising their skills'. In the current research structural reform through the establishment of the division of allied health organisational model and a new executive-level director of allied health position was also an important element through which entrepreneurial professionalism could be mobilised. The importance of structural reform in this study of allied health professions adds to the stock of work supporting the emergence of new organisational forms as an important factor in understanding the nature of entrepreneurialism in public sector health professions.

Entrepreneurial professionalism in the Australian allied health professions could be perceived as a story of engagement with NPM-styled reforms. However, behind the veil of apparent engagement is a complex story of resistance through the mastery of the instruments of change and their appropriation to shape a professionally driven agenda to reconstitute the nature of professionalism. In part this was possible because the allied health managing professional was not a neophyte manager at the time of encountering the reform agenda. This pre-existing managerial experience, together with the first ever opportunity to form their own self-managed divisions, provided resources on which they could manoeuvre in relation to discourses appealing for more business-like and enterprising practice.

Note
[1] Australian Research Council funding for this research project is gratefully acknowledged, as is supplementary funding from The University of Queensland, Research Fellowship Scheme. The assistance of Nicole Shepherd and Dr Sharon Mickan on data assembly, analysis and presentation is also acknowledged.

References

Aldridge, M. (1996) 'Dragged to market: being a profession in the postmodern world', *British Journal of Social Work*, vol 26, pp 177-94.

Borthwick, A.M. (2000) 'Challenging medicine: the case of podiatric surgery', *Work, Employment & Society*, vol 14, no 2, pp 369-83.

Boyce, R.A. (1997) 'Health sector reform and professional power, autonomy and culture: the case of the Australian allied health professions', in R. Hugman, M. Peelo and K. Soothill (eds) *Concepts of care: Developments in health and social welfare*, London: Arnold, pp 74-101.

Boyce, R.A. (2001) 'Organisational governance systems in allied health services: a decade of change', *Australian Health Review*, vol 24, no 1, pp 22-36.

Boyce, R.A. (2004) 'The allied health professions in transition', in M. Clinton (ed) *Management in the Australian health care industry* (3rd edition), Frenchs Forest, NSW: Pearson Education Australia, pp 164-87.

Boyce, R.A. (2006a) 'Using organisation as a strategic resource to build identity and influence', in R. Jones and F. Jenkins (eds) *Managing and leading in the allied health professions*, Oxford: Radcliffe Publishing, pp 85-9.

Boyce, R.A. (2006b) 'Emerging from the shadow of medicine: allied health as a "profession community" subculture', *Health Sociology Review*, vol 15, no 5, pp 520-34.

Braithwaite, J. and Westbrook, M. (2005) 'Rethinking clinical organisational structures: an attitude survey of doctors, nurses and allied health staff in clinical directorates', *Journal of Health Services Research and Policy*, vol 10, no 1, pp 10-17.

Burrows, R. (1991) *Deciphering the enterprise culture: Entrepreneurship, petty capitalism and the restructuring of Britain*, London: Routledge.

Calnan, M., Silvester, S., Manley, G. and Taylor-Gooby, P. (2000) 'Doing business in the NHS: exploring dentists' decisions to practise in the public and private sectors', *Sociology of Health and Illness*, vol 22, no 6, pp 742-64.

Causer, G. and Exworthy, M. (1998) 'Professionals as managers across the public sector', in M. Exworthy and S. Halford (eds) *Professionals and the new managerialism in the public sector*, Buckingham: Open University Press, pp 83-101.

Dent, M. (2003) 'Managing doctors and saving a hospital: irony, rhetoric and actor-networks', *Organization*, vol 10, no 1, pp 107-27.

Dent, M. and Whitehead, S. (2002) 'Introduction: configuring the "new" professional', in M. Dent and S. Whitehead (eds) *Managing professional identities*, London: Routledge, pp 1-18.

Du Gay, P. (1993) 'Entrepreneurial management in the public sector', *Work, Employment & Society*, vol 7, no 4, pp 643-8.

Ennew, C., Feighan, T. and Whynes, D. (1998a) 'Entrepreneurial activity in the public sector: evidence from UK primary care', in P. Taylor-Gooby (ed) *Choice and public policy*, Houndmills: Macmillan, pp 42-61.

Ennew, C., Whynes, D., Jolleys, J. and Robinson, P. (1998b) 'Entrepreneurship and innovation among GP fundholders', *Public Money and Management*, vol 18, no 1, pp 59-64.

Exworthy, M. and Halford, S. (eds) (1998) *Professionals and the new managerialism in the public sector*, Buckingham: Open University Press.

Flynn, R. (1998) 'Managerialism, professionalism and quasi-markets', in M. Exworthy and S. Halford (eds) *Professionals and the new managerialism in the public sector*, Buckingham: Open University Press, pp 18-36.

Foucault, M. (1991) 'Governmentality', in G. Burchell, C. Gordon and P. Miller (eds) *The Foucault effect: Studies in governmentality*, Hemel Hempstead: Harvester Wheatsheaf, pp 89-104.

Fournier, V. (1999) 'The appeal to "professionalism" as a disciplinary mechanism', *Sociological Review*, vol 47, no 2, pp 280-307.

Fournier, V. (2000) 'Boundary work and the (un)making of the professions', in N. Malin (ed) *Professionalism, boundaries and the workplace*, London: Routledge, pp 67-86.

Fournier, V. and Grey, C. (1999) 'Too much, too little and too often: a critique of du Gay's analysis of enterprise', *Organization*, vol 6, no 1, pp 107-28.

Gleeson, D. and Shain, F. (1999) 'Managing ambiguity: between markets and managerialism − case study of "middle" managers in further education', *Sociological Review*, vol 47, no 3, pp 461-90.

Harrison, S. and Dowswell, G. (2002) 'Autonomy and bureaucratic accountability in primary care: what English general practitioners say', *Sociology of Health and Illness*, vol 24, no 2, pp 208-26.

Hood, C. (1991) 'A public management for all seasons?', *Public Administration*, vol 69, no 1, pp 3-19.

Hood, C. (1995) 'The "new public management" in the 1980s: variations on a theme', *Accounting, Organizations and Society*, vol 20, no 2/3, pp 93-109.

Kitchener, M. (2000) 'The "bureaucratisation" of professional roles: the case of clinical directors in UK hospitals', *Organization*, vol 7, no 1, pp 129-54.

Larkin, G. (2002) 'The regulation of the professions supplementary to medicine', in J. Allsop and M. Saks (eds) *Regulating the health professions*, London: Sage Publications, pp 120-33.

Mays, N. and Pope, C. (1997) *Speech and language therapy services and management in the internal market: A national survey*, London: King's Fund Publishing.

Moran, M. (1998) 'Explaining the rise of the market in health care', in W. Ranade (ed) *Markets and health care: A comparative analysis*, London: Longman, pp 17-33.

Øvretveit, J.A. (1992) *Therapy services: Organisation, management and autonomy*, Reading: Harwood Academic Publishers.

Pollitt, C. (1990) *The new managerialism and the public services: The Anglo-American experience*, Oxford: Basil Blackwell.

Powell, M. and Barnett, P. (2001) 'The transformation of an organizational field: institutional pressures and organizational entrepreneurs', Paper presented to the All-Academy Symposium, Academy of Management Annual Conference, Washington, DC, 3-8 August.

Richardson, S. and Cullen, J. (2000) 'Autopsy of change: contextualising entrepreneurial and accounting potential in the NHS', *Financial Accountability and Management*, vol 16, no 4, pp 353-72.

Rowe, P.A., Boyce, R.A., Boyle, M.V. and O'Reilly, K. (2004) 'A comparative analysis of entrepreneurial approaches within public healthcare organisations', *Australian Journal of Public Administration*, vol 63, no 2, pp 16-30.

Thornton, P.H. (1999) 'The sociology of entrepreneurship', *Annual Review of Sociology*, vol 25, pp 19-46.

Whittington, R., McNulty, T. and Whipp, R. (1994) 'Market-driven change in professional services: problems and processes', *Journal of Management Studies*, vol 31, no 6, pp 829-45.

Willis, E. (1989) *Medical dominance: The division of labour in the Australian health care*, Sydney: Allen and Unwin.

Part Two
Drivers and barriers to integration: health
policies and professional development

SIX

Collaborative care and professional boundaries: maternity care in Canada[1]

Ivy Lynn Bourgeault and Elizabeth Darling

Introduction

There is a growing interest in collaborative models of healthcare – or what has alternatively been referred to as 'interprofessionalism' – as a means to address a range of concerns within healthcare systems, not the least of which are shortages of healthcare professionals (DH, 2000; Institute of Medicine, 2003; Health Council of Canada, 2005). Collaborative models of practice are viewed as an important tool for increasing the flexibility of the health labour force. In a recently released report on health human resources in Canada it is argued that 'bringing together physicians and other health professionals to work in teams can be an important part of the solution to challenges such as access to care, wait times for patients, shortages and burn out for professionals' (Task Force Two, 2006, p iv). This reflects the broader view that increased interprofessional collaboration can address human resource shortages both by using existing resources more efficiently and by making the provision of care less demanding on practitioners, thereby improving retention. This has been particularly salient in rural areas where these problems are experienced most acutely (McNair, 2005).

These trends raise a host of issues related to the management of professional boundaries and professional jurisdiction. In a previous article we examined the cases of primary and mental healthcare in Canada and the US in terms of how they revealed the structural embeddedness of medical dominance (Bourgeault and Mulvale, 2006). In this chapter, we seek to look beyond the structural features of the medical profession – or medical dominance – to examine how features of other health professions can also prove to be barriers to collaborative care. We focus on the case of maternity care in Canada, and the province of Ontario more specifically. This case is particularly interesting in light of the relative newness of the midwifery profession to the maternity care division of labour, the rapid changes occurring in maternity care human resources (particularly for intrapartum care) and extensive political and financial support that presently exists for collaborative initiatives in Canada.

Interprofessionalism and professional boundaries

The term 'interprofessionalism' has often been referred to in the literature as synonymous with teamwork or collaboration (Finch, 2000). Several authors have described the attributes of successful models of collaboration with much of this discussion focusing on micro-level factors pertaining to the relationships between the individuals involved (Stapleton, 1998; Rogers, 2003; Anderson, 2005a, 2005b). For example, many articles focus on the culture of interprofessionalism that needs to be created instead of the uniprofessionalism, or the 'silo' mentality, that often persists (Crozier, 2003; Bleakely et al, 2006, Mitchel et al, 2006; see also Pahor, this volume). Others have examined through in-situ conversational analysis the embodied and embedded interactional organisation and dynamics of teamwork (Hindmarsh and Pilnick, 2002).

In addition to these cultural, interactional and attitudinal features are institutional policy factors and broader structural influences on teamwork that Doel (2002, p 170) refers to as 'Berlin walls and garden fences'. One of the key structural influences on collaborative care is the hierarchical nature of the healthcare division of labour. Lichtenstein and colleagues (2004), for example, found that it was the lack of, or the suppression of, full participation among the lower-status members of the healthare team in particular that led to dysfunction. Similarly, Cott (1998) has identified that the unequal power or status of members of long-term care teams makes collaborative teamwork difficult to accomplish because these members remain alienated from the team's decision-making process.

Our interest in this chapter is not so much on the internal workings of maternity care teams, but how these collaborative arrangements are developed in the first instance. We expand our frame of reference beyond the macro level of analysis we undertook in the primary and mental healthcare cases (Bourgeault and Mulvale, 2006) and critically examine the range of factors both promoting and impeding collaborative care models.

Methods and conceptual framework

A multi-method, qualitative approach was employed in this investigation. Data sources included documents from the published academic literature (for instance, secondary sources) and the grey literature (for instance, primary source policy documents, government reports and reports by various stakeholder groups) pertaining to collaborative maternity care in Canada. These were complemented with a series of interviews with key professional and policy stakeholders involved in these decision-making and implementation processes. The analysis of these documents was ongoing throughout the study and served as a basis for the identification of key informants to be interviewed, the questions they would be asked and the development of a preliminary list of barriers to and facilitators of collaborative maternity care we would investigate further.

Interviews were conducted with a total of 34 key informants to explore their views on the factors affecting collaborative maternity care in their jurisdiction (see Table 6.1). Participants were selected through purposive sampling to ensure that key stakeholder positions were represented. The interviews were largely conducted with informants in the province of Ontario but also with national representatives. All interviews followed a semi-structured guide, were conducted by telephone and lasted between 30 and 60 minutes. The initial interview guide focused on questions about the process and factors influencing the decision of who provides what forms of maternity care in their particular area. Structured probes were also included to highlight the influence of different structural, organisational and community-level factors.

Table 6.1: Interview participants by profession and location

	Obstetricians	Family physicians	Midwives	Other[a]
Urban	4	4	4	7
Rural	3	3	4	5
Total	7	7	8	12

Note: [a] Includes anaesthetists, managers and representatives of medical and midwifery regulatory authorities and professional associations.

The interviews were tape-recorded and transcribed and along with key segments from the documents were analysed thematically. In some cases themes emerged directly in response to our interview questions while others emerged from the iterative review process between the documents and the interviews. The rich array of factors raised by our informants and from the documents not only from this case study, but also from our examination of collaborative teams in primary and mental healthcare, led to the development of a conceptual framework (see Table 6.2).

The factors that influence collaborative practice at the micro level include interpersonal relations between team members and any previous experience team members have had working with interdisciplinary teams. Factors at the meso level include the existence of institutional arrangements that either foster or hinder collaborative practice. The broader, macro factors include the influence of regulations around scopes of practice and economic factors, which encompasses both coverage of services (public or private) provided by different potential team members and remunerative models, such as salary or fee-for-service. Liability issues – which cross economic and regulatory domains – are also influential at the macro level.

In the sections that follow we present some of the barriers and facilitators to collaborative maternity care in Canada at these various levels. We begin first, however, with a brief background description of the providers of maternity care in Canada.

Table 6.2: Conceptual model of factors influencing collaborative maternity care

Level	Factors	Details
Micro	Pre-existing relationships	Interprofessional relationships predating collaborative initiative
	Shared desire to address local needs	Common goals of addressing human resource shortages or improving work/life balance are motivators to collaborate
	Philosophy of care	Shared philosophy may decrease apprehensions but also increase a sense of competition; philosophical differences may be a barrier, but respect for differences may be sufficient
Meso	Local human resources	Mix of providers in community; sufficient workload to make practice viable while allowing work/life balance
	Community	Birth rate and needs for maternity care
	Hospitals	Hospital privileges; hospital policies re: transfers; hospital commitment to maternity services
Macro	Economics	Funding models; different funding pools for medical doctors (MDs) and midwives
	Liability	MDs' concern that they are liable for the 'risky' practices of midwives
	Regulation	Requirements of midwifery model of practice; differences in scope of practice

Providers of maternity care in Canada

The key maternity care providers in the Canadian context are physicians – both generalists and specialists – pregnant women are able to access the latter group directly without referral. Only recently – for instance, in 1994 in the province of Ontario – has the option of midwives been made available to some Canadian women. Midwives have been integrated as autonomous primary care providers who provide comprehensive prenatal and intrapartum care to women with uncomplicated pregnancies and births, and care for both the mother and baby until six weeks postpartum (Bourgeault, 2006). Recent figures (2000) indicate that midwives attend approximately 1% of all births in Canada whereas family physicians attend 39% and obstetricians 60% (CIHI, 2004). In the province of Ontario where midwifery has been integrated for over 10 years, midwives attend 7% of births but family physicians only 18% and obstetricians 75%.

These statistics mask some disturbing trends, specifically that there is a looming – and in many rural areas existing – crisis in maternity care. Many physicians, specialist and generalists alike, have been reducing their involvement in the practice of obstetrics due to a variety of reasons, including lifestyle considerations. The small increase in the role of midwives in the provision of maternity care has been insufficient to make up these differences. As a result, the few remaining maternity providers have much higher volume practices, which may result in burnout and an overall unsustainable situation. It is within this context that the push for collaborative models of maternity care has been introduced.

Micro-level influences on collaborative maternity care

Pre-existing relationships

It is not surprising that motivation at the level of individual practitioners to collaborate with other professionals is more likely if positive relationships have already been established. Interviewees involved with a proposal for an integrated pregnancy service described positive interprofessional relationships between maternity care providers. The importance of being familiar with how others work was also identified as the basis for mutual trust. One family physician identified the following to be important in the interactions between obstetricians and family physicians:

> 'There are consultants you work with a million times and they basically know my skill set and … have a comfort with where I blow the whistle and say help, I need your help. Whereas the people who don't know me, you know, obviously are going to behave differently until they get to know me. So it's a question of the relationship and how well you know each other.' (Urban family physician #3)

When trust and respect have already been established, there are likely to be fewer concerns about interprofessional collaboration (see also Calnan and Rowe, and Pahor, this volume).

Desire to address local challenges

Another important factor that can motivate collaboration is a shared desire among individual practitioners to address local maternity care challenges. The primary challenge may be seen as a human resource shortage, or as a need to create call models that allow practitioners to achieve a desired work/life balance. As one family physician described, the current focus on collaborative practice is directed at figuring out how to 'meet women's needs and meet health care providers' needs so that people don't burn out, so that people are able to sustain the practice of maternity care' (urban family physician #3). Other research in Ontario and

Canada has further identified that local leaders or champions of collaborative care are important in moving from a shared desire among local practitioners to address challenges towards a functioning collaborative practice (Anderson, 2005a, 2005b; Rogers et al, 2006).

Philosophy of care

Differences in the philosophy of care of nursing, midwifery and medicine have been identified as a barrier to interprofessional collaboration in interviews with Ontario care providers (Belle Brown et al, 2006). Philosophy of care is often seen as an attribute of a profession's culture, but it would be an oversimplification to assume that an individual's philosophy of care is entirely defined by their profession. Variation in philosophy within professions exists, and when different professionals share a common philosophy, collaboration is more likely to be seen as desirable. Much of the discussion of philosophy of care focused on how differences in philosophy can be a barrier. Several interviewees identified areas where the philosophy of midwives and physicians may differ. This is how one midwife described some of the fundamental aspects of the philosophy of midwifery:

> 'It is a paradigm which recognises that fundamentally birth is normal. That, and that we recognise that the woman needs to be in charge of her body and the primary decision maker about the health of herself and her family, and has the right to have safe care that provides her with the power to choose.' (Rural midwife #2)

Midwives in Ontario are required to provide informed choice, which involves providing clients with thorough information about available options and then supporting the client's preferred option. Medicine has traditionally used a more authoritarian model of decision making in which the physician is viewed as an expert and recommends the best course of action for the patient. The medical model of decision making has gradually been altered by the discourse on informed consent, which has clarified that patients must be provided with a substantial amount of information before they provide consent. Within maternity care, the emphasis on family-centred or woman-centred care has also influenced the importance physicians place on supporting patient choice. In practice, there are variations both in how midwives provide informed choice and in how physicians provide informed consent. In some settings, midwives experience frustration at physicians' understanding of informed choice, while in others, similarity of approach makes this issue less of a concern. Another issue that is related to informed choice is variation in what is seen to be an acceptable level of risk. This issue was identified in focus groups held as part of a Canadian study researching multidisciplinary collaborative maternity care models (Anderson, 2005a).

Midwives are required by the College of Midwives of Ontario to support the choices their clients make. When clients make choices that involve higher levels of risk, this can affect other caregivers' perceptions of midwives. One midwife described comments from an obstetrician colleague and her reaction:

'Recently one obstetrician [said] … that midwives' … first concern is the woman's experience and then the next concern is safety, and that obstetricians are concerned about the safety of the experience and then … the experience of the woman is down the road. And you know, I don't think it's as cut-and-dry like that.' (Rural midwife #2)

In one community, a physician described reluctance to collaborate with the midwife because of discomfort among the family physicians with the midwife's willingness to tolerate potentially complicated circumstances. Other aspects of philosophy seen to be held in common with the midwife were actually cited by this physician as reasons that collaboration was unnecessary:

'We've got a very family-centred maternity care. I mean we've got … a low epidural rate because the physicians and nurses are so supportive of the patients that we've got … just wonderful outcomes here from all the touchy-feely good stuff too, and we're not sure how the midwife can improve on that.... So I've nothing against midwives … I think she has a role but I just see in our particular setting that it's not one that I think she can necessarily add to.' (Rural family physician #4)

Ultimately, in this case, the desire of family physicians to serve the same clients that midwives attract led this physician to interpret the commonalities of family physicians and midwives as a threat rather than an opportunity to collaborate. This suggests that a shared philosophy of care is not a sufficient condition to motivate collaboration. In one Ontario community where physicians and midwives work collaboratively, an understanding that different patients have different wants and needs was identified as an important basis for successful collaboration. Another factor identified was mutual respect between professionals (Jones, 2006). Together, these factors may be enough to overcome differences in philosophy of care among professionals seeking to collaborate.

Meso-level influences on collaborative maternity care

Local human resources

A shortage of maternity care providers is likely to be a strong motivating factor for a community to consider a collaborative care model. As a midwife involved in the integrated pregnancy service proposal put it, 'the purpose of the exercise was to answer the obstetrical care provider crisis here' (rural midwife #4). When there are a limited number of care providers in a community, the heavy workload can be a motivator to ensure that human resources are used efficiently. Creating alternative models is also seen as a way not just to retain but also to attract new practitioners. These were the driving factors in the creation of one collaborative practice.

Another influential factor is the demographics of the existing healthcare providers. Both age and gender may impact how practitioners work. Several interviewees identified changes in physician work patterns that they believe reflect generational differences that might have been led by changes in gender balance, or perhaps are simply masked by gender:

> 'When I think of the doctors who were near retirement when I was doing my residency, many of them had done one-on-one call for years where they followed all their patients, did their own deliveries and so forth ... many of them didn't see very much of their families. I think that now probably my generation and the new graduating residents probably even more so are saying "I want to practise a high standard of medicine. I'm going to be responsible to my patients. But I am also responsible to myself and my family. And I have to achieve a balance here." And that's definitely having an impact with bigger and bigger call groups [with] more flexible care schedules so they can have time off for non-medical interests and for their families.' (Rural obstetrician #1)

Community needs

The size of a community and the number of births occurring within it are probably the most significant attributes of a community affecting the possibility for interprofessional collaboration. The influence of these factors is closely tied to the existing mix of providers in the community. In smaller communities if there is already a reasonable-sized group of family physicians providing obstetrical care and sharing call, they may not want to redistribute births to support the practice of a midwife (Anderson, 2005a, 2005b). In one small community where a group of family physicians worked out a model that provides good continuity for women and limited call for physicians, adding a midwife would dramatically alter the situation: 'I think if we did have a midwife, she would have to assume all of the obstetrical care in order to make it viable for her' (rural family physician #2).

In these types of communities, even if there is a shortage of intrapartum care providers, there may not be enough births for a full-time midwife. For collaborative practice to work in these settings, it was suggested that the midwife might also provide other related services such as prenatal classes, breastfeeding support and well-baby and well-woman care. These kinds of expansions to the current role of the midwife are consistent with the midwives' philosophy and therefore are less controversial for midwives than higher-risk procedures such as vacuum extraction, intubation or ordering inductions.

In communities where there are a greater number of births occurring, there are still challenges in finding a balance between sufficient workload and sufficient time off-call. In 2004 and 2005, obstetricians in Ontario attended an average of 215 births per year, while family physicians attended an average of 19 births per year (Lofsky and Adamson, 2006). A full-time midwife attends 40 births as the primary caregiver. In small- to medium-sized communities the addition or loss of one obstetrician can have a significant impact on the number of births available. This can lead to tensions between professions if any group is left feeling that there are not sufficient births available to support an adequate-sized call group. When remuneration is on a fee-for-service or course-of-care basis, these tensions are more likely to arise. One midwife described this situation in her hospital:

> 'We spoke just very informally to some of our obstetrician colleagues and said, "you know, there is this upcoming crisis looming and insufficient potential obstetricians in the long term. What do you think about midwives offering to cover shifts in terms of doing low risk births? Let's say overnight the obstetricians only had to be called for the actual consultation on complex cases." And they said well they earn their money to make it worthwhile for them being on call by doing those low-risk deliveries.' (Midwifery key informant #10)

In general, in large communities there are enough practitioners available to create adequately sized uni-professional call groups and thus interprofessional collaboration is less likely to arise out of the desire to create models that support less on-call time.

Hospitals

Both midwives and physicians in Ontario must apply for privileges at a hospital in order to attend births there. In a recent survey, privileges were more frequently perceived as a barrier to interprofessional collaboration by midwife educators (about two thirds) than by physician educators (less than one third) (Babies Can't Wait Project, 2006). The funding agreement for midwives in Ontario effectively caps the number of births a midwife can attend each year, so midwifery hospital birth numbers can be capped simply by limiting the number of midwives who are granted privileges. In some cases, restrictions on hospital privileges are driven by hospital administration due to funding issues for nursing care. Lack of hospital privileges makes collaboration between midwives and physicians in a community impossible.

Once a physician or midwife has hospital privileges, obstetrical department policies may influence how they are able to work. The scope of midwifery practice is laid out in detail by the College of Midwives of Ontario but department policies may further restrict this. Hospital limitations on the full scope of midwifery practice can compound existing constraints on midwives' ability to work in partnership with family physicians. Hospital policies may also limit the work that family physicians are able to do. Restrictions on the scope of either midwives or family physicians increase the need for consultations, mainly with obstetricians, who in some hospitals are likely to have the greatest amount of say in what these restrictions are. As one midwife describes:

> 'Fortunately, in [community B] the obstetricians are busy. So quite frankly they're not interested in transferring care for every woman that needs augmentation and an epidural. They don't need the income from it, where in [community C] there's a sense that there's an overall kind of lack of births to go around…. So one of their vested interests in maintaining a high level of transfer of care is that they get income from it.' (Rural midwife #1)

Finally, hospitals influence the opportunities for collaborative care models through their commitment to maintaining obstetrical services. In one community where midwives considered how they might collaborate in order to maintain a dwindling maternity service, the hospital administration's lack of a strong vision to maintain maternity care eventually led to the closure of the birthing unit. Funding issues, particularly the cost of ensuring that the available care and technology is up to date, may play a role in the decisions small hospitals make about maintaining obstetrical services.

Macro-level influences on collaborative maternity care

Funding

Differences in funding mechanisms were frequently cited by interviewees as a barrier to collaborative practice between maternity care providers. In addition to funding for physician and midwifery services coming from separate ministerial branches, the models of remuneration are different. Most physicians providing maternity care services work on a fee-for-service basis, and as one of our informants explained, 'fee for service doesn't fit well with the midwifery model of funding which is currently on a course of care basis' (midwifery key informant #10). In two separate situations where maternity care providers took the initiative to develop proposals for integrated maternity care, funding was identified as one of the two main barriers that eventually prevented physicians and midwives from sharing caseload. In other settings, differences in models of remuneration have prevented practitioners from beginning to explore how they might work together.

Changes to funding were presented as an important aspect of solving the maternity care crisis and retaining practitioners as well as enabling collaboration. Barriers to changing funding models were perceived to exist at several different levels. Some practitioners felt that the government was not willing to come up with solutions to enable interprofessional collaboration that increase costs, such as funding on-call work. It was also noted that physicians providing obstetrical services essentially compete with other physicians for their share of the fee-for-service funding pool, and the priorities of maternity care providers for change may not always be well represented in overall fee negotiations by provincial medical associations who may 'have their own agendas' (urban obstetrician #3).

Liability

Concerns surrounding the liability implications of interprofessional collaboration are another significant barrier. In a survey of educators of future maternity care providers, the barrier to interprofessional collaboration most frequently cited by obstetrician educators was liability (Babies Can't Wait Project, 2006). Physicians believe that if they collaborate with non-physicians they will be considered the most responsible care provider, and therefore will be most liable: 'Our insurance or malpractice membership ... has repeatedly said "you know, watch out for these integrated models because you're medico-legally going to be vulnerable"' (urban obstetrician #3).

This is despite midwives having their own liability insurance. One midwife noted that when midwives in her community were first integrating into the hospital they perceived reluctance from obstetricians to consult, which she attributed to concerns about liability. Once the obstetricians became familiar with the midwives' clinical decision making the relationships became very positive. This suggests that the issue of liability and interprofessional collaboration may be perceived as less of a concern by practitioners who know and respect each other's clinical work than by those who have had little interaction with each other. As a result of initiatives by the Canadian Association of Midwives there has been some work carried out to address these concerns with medical and midwifery liability insurers. While there is yet to be a sweeping endorsement of interprofessional collaboration, these two insurers have been working on a joint statement to address questions of liability when physicians and midwives work together.

Regulation

The other most commonly cited barrier to collaboration between physicians and midwives was the regulations governing midwives' scope and model of practice. Several interviewees identified that current differences between the scopes of practice for midwives and family physicians would make it difficult for these two groups to share call for intrapartum care, particularly in the absence of obstetrical back-up. In other communities physicians see midwives as an obvious choice to fill gaps that currently exist: 'Finding assistants is often very difficult and it seems kind of silly when you have a midwife sitting right there who is fully able to assist and isn't allowed to do it' (rural obstetrician #1).

Potential areas for an expanded midwifery scope that were identified by interviewees included vacuum delivery, ordering oxytocin for augmentation and induction of labour, assisting at Caesarean sections, neonatal intubation, prescription of contraceptives and basic gynaecologic care to healthy non-pregnant women. The issue of an expanded midwifery scope was strongly tied to a consensus that the needs of rural and remote communities differ from those in urban areas. Both what is seen as necessary and what is seen as acceptable depend on location. Maternity care being available as close to home as possible was also highlighted as important. This idea has previously been the basis for training family physicians in advanced maternity skills including Caesarean section (Iglesias et al, 1998).

In addition to issues with scope were concerns around the regulated model of midwifery practice. The College of Midwives of Ontario requires midwives to provide continuity of care, which is defined as midwifery care available 24 hours a day throughout pregnancy from a group of no more than four primary caregivers, and to provide choice of birthplace. The College also requires two midwives to be in attendance at births except in unusual situations (for instance, solo practices). Several sources identified these aspects of the midwifery model of practice as potential barriers to collaboration. Physicians and midwives in one small city in Ontario created a proposal for an integrated pregnancy service in which midwives and family physicians would provide care to low-risk women and share call, and care for high-risk women would be provided by obstetricians. The proposed model challenged the principles of continuity of care, choice of birthplace and two midwives at a birth, which proved to be a barrier in moving forward.

Midwives themselves have registered concern about the limitations of the current model in discussions about the place of midwives within the healthcare system (Tyson, 2001). There is a desire among many midwives for midwifery to play a central role in maternity care and be part of the solution to the current human resource crisis (Cameron and Hutton, 2001). Despite concerns that have been raised about the potential impact of collaboration on midwives' autonomy and their ability to remain true to their core values, many midwives are willing to collaborate, especially when it can make a difference to the services available in their community:

> 'The issue is I don't necessarily want to … do vacuum or intubation but if it is necessary … to keep obstetrics [in my community] then … do I need to do shared care with the doc? Can I help him out so that he doesn't burn out? So those are the things that we're sort of talking about.' (Rural midwife #3)

The Ontario Medical Association has also criticised the College of Midwives of Ontario for not supporting intraprofessional care as an overall approach to care (OMA, 2006). The College of Midwives of Ontario has proceeded cautiously in approving changes to the model to enable more interprofessional collaboration.

To date one pilot project involving collaboration between midwives and a nurse practitioner has been approved.

Discussion

In sum, we find many similar barriers and facilitators to collaborative maternity care that many others have noted, particularly at the level of interprofessional relationships and institutional culture, with some nuances around different philosophies of care. It is at the structural level, however, that this case helps to uncover some key factors previously unexamined in the literature. As we noted at the outset, one of the positions we wanted to elucidate in this chapter is that it is not only the structural features of the medical profession, or what we refer to elsewhere as the 'structural embeddedness' of medical dominance, that has proven to be a barrier to collaborative practice arrangements (Bourgeault and Mulvale, 2006), but also the particular structural features of the midwifery profession – in this case their regulated model of care. These structural features were not intended to put up barriers to collaborative practice but rather to protect what was seen when these regulations were put into place – and in some cases is still seen – as a vulnerable profession. The caution that midwives have exercised in proceeding with collaborative arrangements is also illustrative of a desire to not compromise their unique philosophy of birth as a normal, non-medicalised process (Van Wagner, 2004).

Similar concerns with the dilution of a non-medical model of practice were also salient in the cases of primary and mental healthcare we examined both in Canada and the US, but the non-medical providers in these cases – primarily nurse practitioners, physician assistants and psychologists – were less likely to have the kind of protective legislation for their model of practice than afforded to the midwifery profession (Bourgeault, 2006). This difference can be explained in part because of the greater success of Ontario midwives vis-à-vis state policy makers, but also because of the greater openness of the medical profession to work collaboratively in (or alternatively the desire to control) primary and mental healthcare than maternity care (Bourgeault, 2005). Thus, it is not only the direct impact of medical dominance that suppresses the full participation of all team members, but an extension of arguments made by previous authors on collaborative or team-based care suggests that it also indirectly influences the desire to even participate in such ventures in the first place.

Note

[1] Funding for this research was provided by the Canadian Institutes for Health Research and the Faculty of Social Science at McMaster University, Canada.

References

Anderson, M. (2005a) 'Focus group report', Discussion paper prepared for The Multidisciplinary Collaborative Primary Maternity Care Project, Ottawa, www.mcp2.ca/english/documents/FinalIntvwReptMar05.pdf

Anderson, M. (2005b) 'Interview report', Discussion paper prepared for the Multidisciplinary Collaborative Primary Care Project, Ottawa, www.mcp2.ca/english/documents/FinalIntvwReptMar05.pdf

Babies Can't Wait Project (2006) 'A study of future maternity care providers and their educators', Paper presented to the Ideas into Action Toronto, Consensus Building Workshop, Toronto, Ontario, 25-26 May 2006.

Belle Brown, J., Bickford, J., Stewart, M., Freeman, T. and Kasperski, J. (2006) 'Babies can't wait: provider qualitative interviews', Paper presented to the Ideas into Action Toronto, Consensus Building Workshop, Toronto, Ontario, 25-26 May 2006.

Bleakley, A., Boyden, J., Hobbs, A., Walsh, L. and Allard, J. (2006) 'Improving teamwork climate in operating theatres: the shift from multiprofessionalism to interprofessionalism', *Journal of Interprofessional Care*, vol 20, no 5, pp 461-70.

Bourgeault, I.L. (2005) 'Gendered professionalization strategies and the rationalization of health care: midwifery, nurse practitioners, and hospital nurse staffing in Ontario, Canada', *Knowledge, Work and Society*, vol 3, no 1, pp 25-52.

Bourgeault, I.L. (2006) *Push! The struggle for midwifery in Ontario*, Montreal: McGill-Queen's University Press.

Bourgeault, I.L. and Mulvale, G. (2006) 'Collaborative health care teams in Canada and the U.S.: confronting the structural embeddedness of medical dominance', *Health Sociology Review*, vol 15, no 5, pp 481-95.

Cameron, C. and Hutton, E. (2001) 'The maternity care crisis in Canada: what role can midwives play?', *Association of Ontario Midwives Journal*, vol 7, no 1, pp 17-20.

CIHI (Canadian Institute for Health Information) (2004) *Giving birth in Canada: Providers of maternity and infant care*, http://dsp-psd.pwgsc.gc.ca/Collection/H118-25-2004E.pdf

Cott, C. (1998) 'Structure and meaning in multidisciplinary teamwork', *Sociology of Health and Illness*, vol 20, no 6, pp 848-73.

Crozier, K. (2003) 'Interprofessional education in maternity care: shared learning for women-centred care', *International Journal of Sociology and Social Policy*, vol 23, no 4/5, pp 123-38.

DH (Department of Health) (2000) *A health service for all talents: Developing the NHS workforce*, London: The Stationery Office.

Doel, M. (2002) 'Interprofessional working: Berlin walls and garden fences', *Learning in Health and Social Care*, vol 1, no 3, pp 170-1.

Finch, J. (2000) 'Interprofessional education and teamworking: a view from the education providers', *British Medical Journal*, vol 321, pp 1138-40.

Health Council of Canada (2005) *Modernizing the management of HHR in Canada – report from a national summit,* www.phac-aspc.gc.ca/php-psp/pdf/moderniz_the_management_of_health_human_resources_in_canada_e.pdf

Hindmarsh, J. and Pilnick, A. (2002) 'The tacit order of teamwork: collaboration and embodied conduct in anaesthesia', *The Sociological Quarterly,* vol 43, no 2, pp 139-64.

Iglesias, S., Grzybowski, S., Klein, M.C., Gagne, G.P. and Lalonde, A. (1998) 'Joint position paper on rural maternity care, Joint Working Group', *Canadian Family Physician,* vol 44, pp 831-43.

Institute of Medicine (2003) *Health professions education: A bridge to quality,* Washington, DC: The National Academy Press, http://search.nap.edu/books/0309087236/html

Jones, G. (2006) 'Collaborative maternity care: the Winchester experience', Paper presented to the Ideas into Action Toronto, Consensus Building Workshop, Toronto, Ontario, 25-26 May 2006.

Lichtenstein, R., Alexander, J.A., McCarthy, J.F. and Wells, R. (2004) 'Status differences in cross-functional teams: effects on individual member participation, job satisfaction, and intent to quit', *Journal of Health and Social Behavior,* vol 45, no 3, pp 322-35.

Lofsky, S. and Adamson, M. (2006) 'Changing trends in obstetrical physician human resources in Ontario, 1992-2005', Paper presented to the Ideas into Action Toronto, Consensus Building Workshop, Toronto, Ontario, 25-26 May 2006.

McNair, R. (2005) *Breaking down the silos: Interprofessional education and interprofessionalism for an effective rural health care workforce,* www.ruralhealth.org.au/nrhapublic/publicdocs/conferences/8thNRHC/Papers/KN_mcnair,%20ruth.pdf

Mitchell, P.H., Belza, B., Schaad, D.C., Robins, L.S., Gianola, F.J., Odegard, P.S., Kartin, D. and Ballweg, R.A. (2006) 'Working across the boundaries of health professions disciplines in education, research, and service: the University of Washington experience', *Academic Medicine,* vol 81, no 10, pp 891-6.

OMA (Ontario Medical Association) (2006) 'OMA response to the Ontario maternity care expert panel report', *Ontario Medical Review,* vol 73, no 9, p 23.

Rogers, J. (2003) 'Sustainability and collaboration in maternity care in Canada: dreams and obstacles', *Canadian Journal of Rural Medicine,* vol 8, no 3, pp 193-8.

Rogers, J., Roy Sen, A. and Sorbara, L. (2006) 'Integrated maternity care for rural and remote communities', Paper presented to the Ideas into Action Toronto, Consensus Building Workshop, Toronto, Ontario, 25-26 May 2006.

Stapleton, S.R. (1998) 'Team-building: making collaborative practice work', *Journal of Nurse-Midwifery,* vol 43, no 1, pp 12-18.

Task Force Two (2006) *A physician human resource strategy for Canada: Final report,* www.physicianhr.ca/reports/TF2FinalStrategicReport-e.pdf

Tyson, H. (2001) 'The integrity of midwifery in Ontario and its integration into the health care system', *Association of Ontario Midwives Journal,* vol 7, no 1, pp 21-5.

Van Wagner, V. (2004) 'Why legislation? Using regulation to strengthen midwifery', in I.L. Bourgeault, C. Benoit and R. Davis-Floyd (eds) *Reconceiving midwifery*, Montreal: McGill-Queen's University Press, pp 71-90.

SEVEN

Interprofessional relationships: doctors and nurses in Slovenia

Majda Pahor

Introduction

Collaboration of different professional groups is an important dimension of the quality and efficiency of healthcare services that directly impact on patient outcomes. However, the relationships between the two largest professional groups in healthcare – nurses and doctors – have been traditionally hierarchical. In its classical version, professionalism is characterised by strategies of social exclusion, closure and demarcation. In particular, medical 'tribalism' and the interprofessional relationships between doctors and nurses have always been an area of conflict, although these relationships are also subject to general trends of inclusion and participation. Changes in social context – such as democratisation, women's emancipation and higher levels of education – challenge the rigid structure of healthcare systems. New demands on healthcare and citizenship rights create a new need for more collaborative relationships; across countries, professionalism is in a process of transformation towards more inclusive forms (Saks and Kuhlmann, 2006).

This chapter discusses the nurse–doctor relationship in the Slovenian healthcare system. It is argued that options for, and barriers to, collaboration are not only shaped by organisational context and governance structures, they are also embedded in 'culture' and modelled by professional identity and individual attitudes. An important element of changing or sustaining a hierarchical structure of interprofessional relations is the perception that members of these two professional groups hold about themselves and each other. In Slovenia, no systematic 'map' and database exist on interprofessional relationships between nurses and doctors. In 2004, however, both professional associations – the Nurse and Midwifery Organisation of Ljubljana (part of Nurses Association of Slovenia – NAS) and the Slovenian Medical Association (SMA) – agreed to support research into the perceptions that these two professional groups hold about each other and their relationship.

This chapter focuses on the empirical findings of this study. It places the individual perceptions and actor-based changes in the Slovenian healthcare system in the context of the historical formation of Roman Catholic culture and the experiences of centralised bureaucracy of the socialist era. The concept of individualisation and self-determination and the notion of trust (see also Calnan and Rowe, this volume) serve to explore the complexity and cultural embeddedness of professional relationships in healthcare.

Different cultures of doctors and nurses: working together apart

Collaboration in healthcare calls for the participation and more equal relationships of all players involved. It touches on the role of the individual in society and broader societal changes towards 'individualisation'. According to Beck and Beck-Gernsheim (2002), the move of societies towards individualisation is characterised by activity, initiative, flexibility and, above all, knowledge of such practices. Following this argument, individualisation is a precondition for collaboration; it is not possible to develop cooperative relationships without the prior autonomy of individuals. Furthermore, empirical findings highlight that professional autonomy does not hinder collaboration (Rafferty et al, 2001). However, new demands on collaboration do not fit easily into a historically developed culture of medical supremacy and hierarchy in healthcare.

Several studies in different health systems highlight problems in the relationships between nurses and doctors (Walby and Greenwell, 1994; Ryan, 1996; Salvage and Smith, 2000; Aiken et al, 2001; Zwarenstein and Bryant, 2004; San Martin Rodriguez et al, 2005; for a historical analysis see Dingwall et al, 1991). The sources of conflict are complex. Doctors and nurses have different class backgrounds, and gender also matters: the medical profession is traditionally a male profession and nursing a female profession. Differences in education are also relevant, not only in the declared educational objectives, but also in the hidden curriculum. Added to this, nurses and doctors occupy different positions in the organisational structure of healthcare, which often hinders cooperation. Although these sources of conflict cannot be abolished in the near future, new health policies and actor-based changes in the professions and society at large place new pressures on both professional groups to remodel their attitudes and the lines of division in healthcare.

For a long time, the medical profession served as a model for professionalisation and upward social mobility (Freidson, 1994). Within this classic model, professionalism and autonomy were connected in ways that guaranteed the hegemony of the medical profession and the deference of the allied health professions with a higher overall proportion of women. However, in most Western countries the medical profession is struggling to maintain status, while some other health professions, like nursing and midwifery, are striving for upward social mobility (Broadbent, 1998; Blättel-Mink and Kuhlmann, 2003; Bourgeault et al, 2004; Witz and Annandale, 2006). Similar trends can be observed in Slovenia. For instance, research into the social reputation of different professions has revealed interesting shifts since the 1980s: doctors hold the highest position, but the proportion of those who see doctors as highly reputable has decreased slightly (from 86% to 83%), while positive judgements on nurses have increased significantly (from 30% to 46%) (Toš, 2004).

Processes of democratisation and pluralisation of late modern societies have challenged traditional hierarchical relationships, such as the position of women and young people, the roles of different occupational and professional groups and the needs and demands of patients. The classic image of medicine as a male profession is no longer sustainable: taken over the whole spectrum of medical specialties, women are in the majority, especially in Eastern European countries and – to a lesser extent – also in Central Europe (see also Riska and Novelskaite, this volume). The proportion of women is also on the increase in Western countries. Further pressures for change may arise from new health policies that attempt to use the generally positive impact of collaboration as a lever for rationalising organisation and service delivery. For example, a recent Cochrane review highlights that collaboration can improve the outcomes of healthcare (Zwarenstein and Bryant, 2004; see also Wensing et al, 2006): it reduces the number of days spent in hospital and treatment costs, and improves patients' satisfaction and the mutual respect of health professionals (see also Baggs, 2006). Micro-level qualitative studies into collaboration, using observation and in-depth interviews, also indicate a positive overall impact on the quality of care (Soederberg, 1999; Thomas et al, 2003).

One of the consequences of the new pressures for collaboration is manifest in the changes in the educational and training system of health professionals. Analyses of the hidden curriculum of medical and nursing departments reveal working situations that are hierarchical, competitive and disrespectful, where students are sometimes treated in a humiliating manner, leading to the development of separate, sometimes even hostile, subcultures (Essex, 1995; Lempp and Seale, 2004). As a consequence, different health systems have introduced interprofessional learning in undergraduate and postgraduate programmes (Barret et al, 2003; Pollard et al, 2004) and in continuing education (Bateman et al, 2003).

Although the available research points to the benefits of interprofessional care for health systems and individuals, the concept of collaboration is complex and difficult to establish (Kollock, 1998; D'Amour et al, 2005). Drawing on developments in the British National Health Service (NHS), Davies (2000) highlights that collaboration very rarely arises spontaneously, but needs systematic encouragement. Relevant determinants are identified on three levels: system, organisation and interaction (San Martin Rodriguez et al, 2005). Apart from the system characteristics – social, political and cultural factors, including the educational system and values – the most direct influence on interprofessional collaboration may derive from organisational determinants. However, interaction factors matter too, such as readiness to collaborate, trust, communication, mutual respect, self-confidence, power and defences against anxiety (Barret and Keeping, 2005; San Martin Rodriguez et al, 2005).

Furthermore, attitudes towards collaboration are culturally sensitive and can support or hinder collaboration. International comparative studies (for instance, Hojat et al, 2003) show the existence of predominantly hierarchical models of relationships in healthcare teams in some countries and predominantly complementary models in others. In countries where collaboration is more entrenched in the educational system, nurses and doctors also have more positive attitudes towards collaboration. Interestingly, a British study of medical and nursing students points to an even greater interest of nurses in collaboration (Hean et al, 2006). I will come back to this issue later in this chapter.

Taken together, available research indicates that collaboration is not simply a matter of professional governance and organisational change, but must be assessed in its social and cultural context.

The case of Slovenia: crossroads of Central and Eastern Europe with some 'warm winds' in the South

Slovenia has undergone a transition from a one-party political system to democratic pluralism and from a state-centred, socialist economy and welfare system to a market economy. The economic and organisational changes have been discussed intensively in social and health policy, but the cultural and interactional dimensions have so far been ignored. The transformations clearly impact on the healthcare system, but they do not automatically lead to flexibility and more participatory relationships. Instead, hierarchical relationships persist in the health workforce (Klemenc and Pahor, 2001; Klemenc et al, 2003). Although Slovenia has a highly educated health workforce, human resources are not used effectively.

In 2005 a study of the organisational culture of Slovenian hospitals revealed that leadership is directed towards coordination and organisation, and formal rules and order are the primary interest. Where a market culture does exist, it is still based on control, efficacy and productivity and characterised by centralised decision making, competitiveness and an outcome orientation. Slovenian hospitals are therefore dominated by a culture of control rather than a culture of flexibilisation and professional development (Skela-Savič et al, 2006). However, a culture of hierarchy and control is not simply a relic of socialist bureaucracy – which is destined to disappear in the long run.

The concept of social capital, conceptualised as generalised trust, provides an opportunity for a better understanding of the interplay of different cultures and their impact on collaboration (Iglič, 2004; see also Calnan and Rowe, this volume). In Slovenia, social capital is low compared to other European countries, and collaboration and integration inadequate at all levels of the social system. High levels of social capital (more than 60% of the population trust other people) are reported in the Scandinavian countries and the Netherlands, and low levels (around 20%) in Southern and Eastern European countries. Although the level of mutual trust has increased since the mid-1990s, Slovenia remains in the group of low-trust countries (Delhey and Newton, 2003; Iglič, 2004).

The asymmetrical distribution of social capital and its geographical concentration underscores the importance of historical and cultural influences. According to Inglehart (1999), a combination of the Catholic and Communist past is a predictor for low levels of social capital. Slovenia experienced the socialist system for half a century. In former socialist countries the dominant social element was atomism; social exchange worked in instrumental relationships, while generalised reciprocity was limited to the family. At the same time, Slovenia belongs to the cultural and political space of Central Europe. For more than 600 years, it was part of the conservative and very Catholic Habsburg monarchy, where rapid cultural development during the short Protestant era was brutally interrupted.

According to Inglehart (1997), Catholic countries also have lower levels of trust because of the hierarchical social structure, shaped by the Roman Catholic Church. In traditionally Catholic countries, religiosity is connected with value orientations characterised by obedience and subservience. In contrast, the values of freedom, autonomy and self-realisation are connected with equity, tolerance and justice. Countries with more developed post-materialist value orientations show higher levels of altruistic trust, where post-materialism involves valuing self-realisation and tolerance towards the social and natural environment (Inglehart, 1997).

Analysis of the European Values Survey highlights four value orientations in Slovenia – namely traditionalism, materialism, egoistic individualism and sympathetic individualism (Iglič, 2004). There were few European countries with such a clear-cut categorisation of value orientations – besides Slovenia, these included Spain and Italy, and, to a lesser extent, Austria and Belgium, which are all countries with a strong Catholic tradition. A traditional orientation includes religion and obedience; materialism values hard work and thrift; egoistic individualism (which was also predominant in Eastern European countries) values ego-centrism and autonomy; and sympathetic individualism translates as a positive orientation towards others, as well as individual freedom.

Comparing Slovenia with other European countries reveals elements of egoistic individualism and strong traditionalism, in combination with religion and the authoritarian valuing of obedience. The first element might be the result of the socialist era – as it is shared with other Eastern European countries – and the second one might be derived from the Catholic tradition (Inglehart, 1997). Both value systems provoke a number of tensions – and even contradictions – that lead to new demands on collaboration and teamwork in healthcare. It can therefore be assumed that the cultural context of the Slovenian health system creates its own changes in professional identities and attitudes that may either promote or inhibit collaboration.

Attitudes towards interprofessional relations: the empirical investigation

An important element of changing or sustaining the existing structure of nurse–doctor relationships is the perceptions that members of these two professional groups hold about themselves and each other. The findings reported here are based on a larger research programme and a multi-method study comprising a survey and several qualitative studies. A literature review served to develop a model of an 'ideal type' of attitudes related to readiness for, and the possibility of, improved interprofessional collaboration between nurses, nursing assistants and doctors. The assumption was that there is a greater possibility for collaboration if the respondents' answers are close to the ideal type and differences between the three professional groups are small.

A questionnaire study was carried out in order to gather data, comprising the following key questions:

- How do Slovenian doctors, nurses and nursing assistants experience interprofessional relations?
- How do they characterise the relationships?
- How do they assess themselves as communicators and team workers?
- To what extent are they satisfied with the overall work situation?

The questionnaire was divided into three scales – 'experiencing', 'characteristics' and 'communication' – plus a question on workplace satisfaction and demographic characteristics. In addition, two open questions were included: 'what is a health care team?' and 'would you like to comment on the topic of the research study?'. The three scales applied here were developed by the research group at the Faculty of Health and Social Care at the University of the West of England in Bristol in the UK (Pollard et al, 2004). Transferring research instruments from one language and culture to another has its pitfalls; cultural differences between the countries may be reflected in a lack of common expressions and recognisable situations. However, cultural bias was reduced as far as possible.

The first scale, termed 'experiencing interprofessional relations', was designed to measure the subjective aspects of interprofessional relations, following the assumption that individuals may experience the same situation differently. The second scale, 'characteristics of the interprofessional relations', aimed to identify the respondents' judgements on the 'objective' situation of interprofessional relations. Here the assumption was that individuals may assess the general conditions differently from their own experiences, reasoning for example that: 'my own team is okay, we collaborate well, but the situation between nurses and doctors in general is not okay'. The third scale, 'communication and teamwork', aimed to assess whether the respondents perceive themselves as good communicators and team collaborators. This scale was expected to reveal more 'fine-tuned' perceptions of teamwork in the three professional groups. All three scales were tested for reliability using principal component analysis and Cronbach alpha. Both methods showed high internal consistency of the instruments (Cronbach alpha coefficients: 0.876, 0.913 and 0.833 respectively).

Participants in the survey, carried out in May 2005, were selected from among 4,298 members of the Slovenian Medical Association and 12,956 members of the Slovenian Nursing Association. The questionnaire was mailed to a randomised sample, comprising 20% of the population – 800 doctors and 2,646 nurses and nursing assistants. The response rate was 22.3% in the doctors' sample and 19.2%

in the sample of nurses and nursing assistants. In all, 686 questionnaires were returned: 178 from doctors, 261 from nurses and 247 from nursing assistants.

The profiles of the sample reflected, as closely as possible, the population at large. The sample included 58% of female doctors and 42% of male doctors, thus mirroring the gender composition of the Slovenian medical profession. The gender ratio of nurses and nursing assistants was also representative (slightly more than 90% women). In relation to the level of education, our sample was representative of the group of doctors and nurses, but the response rate of the nursing assistants was much lower than for the group as a whole. About half of the respondents worked in hospitals, nearly one third in primary care and the remaining group in diverse health and social care institutions and in private practice.

Before discussing the results, the limitations of the study must be taken into consideration. The overall response rate was low (20%) and the low participation of the nursing assistants, in particular, is a weakness of the study. Furthermore, the research instruments were developed in another culture, a culture, moreover, that might differ from Slovenia more than expected. The study does, however, for the first time, provide important information on prevailing attitudes and judgements with regard to interprofessional relationships in the largest occupational groups drawn from about 700 questionnaires. Furthermore, a large number of the participants in the questionnaire study answered the open questions (562 the first question and 230 the second question). These data, together with nine semi-structured interviews, provide the material for the qualitative analysis in the study.

Variations on a theme: collaboration from the perspective of doctors and nurses

The findings highlight significant differences in the definitions and perceptions of interprofessional relationships between the three professional groups involved in the study. Most importantly, doctors were most satisfied with the situation at the workplace; they reported good experiences overall with interprofessional work with nurses and nursing assistants. They were also positive about the general characteristics of interprofessional relations, and perceived themselves as the best communicators and teamworkers of the three groups. The nursing group – including state registered nurses and nursing assistants – showed broadly similar judgements. However, the judgements differed significantly when it came to the characteristics of interprofessional relations: nurses were more critical than nursing assistants, and less positive about the quality of the relationships involved.

To return to our hypothesis on 'ideal types' and collaboration, doctors come closest to the ideal type of judgements on relations in healthcare. Consequently, doctors predominantly think that the relationships between nurses and doctors are satisfactory.

'It is easy to collaborate, if others do as they are told.'

The results for the first scale (Figure 7.1), which measured the 'experiencing' of interprofessional relations, highlight correlations between positive experiences and high scores for 'understanding of one's professional role' and self-confidence at work with one's own and other professional groups. Negative perceptions correlate with low self-confidence and lack of doctors' respect for the other two groups. For the group of doctors in the study negative experiences are mainly an intraprofessional problem, while relations with doctors are the main source of negative experiences for nurses and nursing assistants.

Qualitative analysis indicates that 'respect' – together with professional knowledge and skills – are perceived as key elements of positive interprofessional relations. For instance, one female doctor stated: 'And when everybody in the team strives for good professional work and respectful relations, there are neither problems with co-workers nor with patients'.

In-depth analysis of the data reveals three levels of respect relevant for interprofessional relations: respect towards other professions, respect towards different levels of education and respect towards the individual. It is important to note, however, that respect was more often mentioned negatively: for instance, underestimation and devaluation of the competencies of other professions, and even lack of respect related to the profession, education, gender and status. Evidence of disrespect not only appeared between professions, but also in intraprofessional relations, especially between nurses and nursing assistants (see also Domajnko et al, 2006).

'We are fine, but they are a problem.'

Differences between the three groups were especially strong in the perception of the 'characteristics' of interprofessional relations. Generally, doctors did not perceive the relationships as a conflictual issue. This points to a lack of critical reflection that may be a result of the dominant role of doctors in healthcare; consequently, pressures for change are low in the medical profession. Nursing assistants were only slightly less satisfied than doctors. Here, the lack of criticism may be a result of their (female) socialisation into acceptance of existing hierarchical relations.

In contrast to doctors and nursing assistants, the nurses perceived the relationships as much more problematic and showed the lowest level of satisfaction with interprofessional relations. The more critical perspective of nurses may be nurtured by the changes in their curriculum over the past decade. It may also be supported by an overall changing self-image of women, especially of the younger generation. The findings indicate that nurses are no longer willing to accept subordination in the healthcare system, and therefore judge interprofessional relationships more critically. However, as mentioned previously, the subsample of nurses who studied in the new programme that started in 1996 was overrepresented, and criticism may thus be more strongly emphasised than in the nursing profession as a whole.

Figure 7.1: Differences in the perception of interprofessional relations

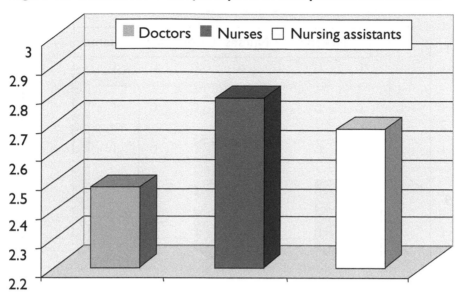

Notes: F=27.30; p=0.000.

Positive perceptions of interprofessional relations – the lower the score, the more positive the perceptions.

Nevertheless, compared to the other two groups, nurses seem to be a driving force for improved collaboration.

Analysis of the variance of the second scale – 'characteristics' – shows that high scores are positively correlated with the item 'respect for another discipline', and low scores with the item 'status hierarchy'. In the latter, the differences between the three professional groups were strongest compared to the other two scales. On the 'communication' scale (Figure 7.2) high scores were positively correlated to the items 'ability of working in group' and 'ability of explaining to co-workers'. Low scores, in contrast, were correlated to the items 'problems of expressing disagreement' and 'inability to express disagreement'. Nurses and nursing assistants, especially, often mentioned problems with taking initiative in the workplace. As already mentioned, however, overall the differences between the professions were low.

The analysis highlights a stronger impact of the profession on the 'characteristics' scale compared to the 'experiencing' and 'communication' scales. This brings into focus a differentiation between the judgements regarding individual situations and the position of the profession in the health workforce as a whole. The items on the scales 'experiencing' and 'communication' were addressed in the first person singular – speaking about 'me' – while the items on the 'characteristics' scale were related to a professional group – speaking about 'them'.

The findings suggest different things with respect to collaboration (Figure 7.3). First, there is a potential for improved interprofessional relations and collaboration:

Figure 7.2: Self-assessment of communication and teamwork skills

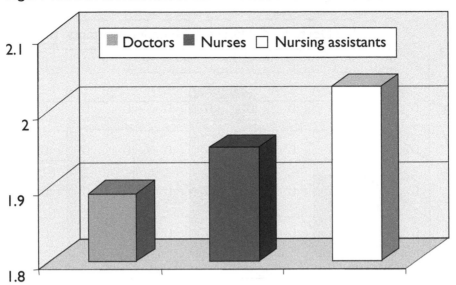

Notes: F=3.125; p=0.045.

Self-assessment of communication and teamwork skills – the lower the score, the more positive the assessment.

the overall work satisfaction is high and the two scales 'experiencing' and 'communication' show broadly similar perceptions in the three groups. Second, the individual work situation is perceived more positively than the collective situation and the potential for collaboration. Third, nurses are more critical about the quality of interprofessional relations and more willing to improve collaboration than doctors.

The 'lived' interprofessional relationships

The potential for collaborative care was further explored in drawing on qualitative analysis (Strauss, 1995). Our interest focused on the observed differences between individual perceptions and more general judgements on collaboration. One topic chosen for in-depth analysis was the individual experience with teamwork; another topic was the definition of the concept of healthcare teams, addressing issues of collaboration, status and hierarchy, respect and the possibility of expressing one's own ideas.

A major finding is that most of the descriptions of the healthcare team were in the conditional form, like 'team should include', indicating that teamwork is not a reality for the majority of the respondents. One respondent, a female nurse, even stated: 'This is something that does not exist in the Slovenian hospitals'. Very few respondents used the first person singular or plural when describing the characteristics of a team. Furthermore, patients were nearly totally absent in

Figure 7.3: Readiness for collaboration between professional groups

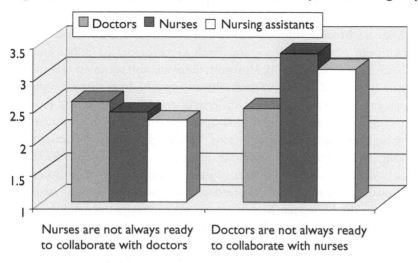

Notes: 'Nurses are not always ready to collaborate with doctors', *F*=4.776; *p*=0.009.
'Doctors are not always ready to collaborate with nurses', *F*=55.396; *p*=0.000.
Figure shows proportion of doctors, nurses and nursing assistants who agree with the statements.

the descriptions of team characteristics, although many respondents mentioned the direct impact of collaboration on patient outcomes.

Content analysis identified 'collaboration' as the key element of teamwork, and six related categories: common goal, common work, autonomy, decision making, communication and values. Collaboration was described as the essential feature of teamwork, and autonomy of the different team members as a precondition for the functioning of teams. Professional autonomy based on knowledge was assumed to reduce hierarchy between the players involved in teamwork and to enable the team to reach the common goal of the well-being of patients and satisfaction of each team member. Further enabling conditions were mentioned, such as a clear division of work and responsibilities, and a shift from traditionally hierarchical patterns of decision making to more democratic procedures. Respondents claimed that decision making should depend on professional knowledge and skills rather than on status. They stressed a need for complementary skills and equality of all team members rather than the delegation of tasks.

Equality was defined as the possibility to express one's opinion and make suggestions from the point of view of the different professions that make up a healthcare team. It is interesting here to take a closer look at the metaphors that were chosen to describe the team. For instance, the team was termed a 'chain with the members as the links'; 'a palace built from mutually supporting stones'; and 'a mosaic picture which would not be perfect if only the merest part was missing'. Similarly, equality of team members was described in terms of 'two-way' communication or the 'enabling exchange of opinions'. Such patterns of communication were perceived to be supported by professional ethics that encourage values like tolerance, respect, openness, trust and mutual help.

The findings are broadly supported by the literature and echo developments in other European countries (Beck and Beck-Gernsheim, 2002; Mickan and Rodgers, 2005; Pethybridge, 2004). However, there are also some aspects specific to the cultural context of the Slovenian healthcare system. In particular, cohesion as a team characteristic was observed in an Australian study (Mickan and Rodgers, 2005), but completely absent in our sample. At the same time, autonomy ranked very high on the agenda in Slovenia. This might reflect the actual stage of establishing collaboration in Slovenian healthcare. Autonomy is linked to individualisation, knowledge and the active participation of different professions. At present, however, only the medical profession possesses the classical attributes of a profession in the Slovenian healthcare system. Consequently, collaboration occurs as a limited option, especially for nurses.

Healthcare teams do exist, but are based – first and foremost – on hierarchy rather than on participatory relationships and the collaboration of team members. This conclusion is supported by findings from the subgroup of professionals that held managerial positions. Under these conditions, collaboration may emerge as a sporadic event or individual experience, but not as a systematic part of the strategy of workforce planning and reorganisation of healthcare.

Conclusion

This chapter has set out to explore the attitudes of nurses, nursing assistants and doctors on interprofessional relations in the Slovenian healthcare system and the potential for collaboration and teamwork. The findings highlight significant differences between the three groups that point to tensions and sources of conflict. At the same time, there are also similarities, like readiness to work in groups, and perceptions of the problems of establishing collaboration and healthcare teams. The respondents from all three professional groups expressed 'respect' for the other disciplines: many doctors stated that they had respect for nurses, as did nurses and nursing assistants for doctors. However, nurses and nursing assistants did not think that doctors respected the nursing profession. But all three groups stated that they understood the professional roles of other groups and all three were aware that hierarchy influences interprofessional relationships.

A number of conclusions can be drawn from the findings. One conclusion is that the two biggest professional groups have obviously reached a situation where they are ready to face their own uncertainties about how healthcare work should be performed, and ready to introduce some changes into the old hierarchical patterns. Readiness for collaboration and the critique of existing hierarchies are strongest in the group of nurses, and nurses may therefore act as a driving force towards collaboration. This situation may be the result of processes of women's emancipation and improved education and training; the changing emphasis on citizenship participation and European policies may also have had an impact.

Another conclusion is that 'Europeanisation' has had no linear impact on professional relationships in healthcare. On the one hand, increasing international collaboration and exchange with North Western Europe has brought new ideas on how healthcare can be governed in Slovenia. On the other hand, very patriarchal relationships and low levels of nursing education that persist in some influential European countries – like Austria and Germany – may have had a negative impact on the transformation of the Slovenian health workforce. The study also highlights the significance of 'culture' in arriving at a better understanding of the governance of healthcare. It underscores the context dependency of professional governance and workforce development. Professional relationships and the options for, and barriers to, collaboration are embedded in the Slovenian culture of Roman Catholic value orientations and the former experiences of hierarchical bureaucracy during the socialist era. Within this historical framework, the observed transformation of interprofessional relationships between doctors and nurses creates its own conditions and dynamics, marked by a generally slow pace of change.

References

Aiken, L.H., Clarke, S.P., Sloane, D.M., Sochalski, J.A., Busse, R., Clarke, H., Giovannetti, P., Hunt, J., Rafferty, A.M. and Shaiman, J. (2001) 'Nurses' reports on hospital care in five countries', *Health Affairs*, vol 20, no 3, pp 43-53.

Baggs, G.J. (2006) 'Overview and summary: partnership and collaboration – what skills are needed?', *Online Journal of Issues in Nursing*, vol 10, no 1, www.nursingworld.org/ojin/topic26/tpc26ntr.htm

Barret, G. and Keeping, C. (2005) 'The processes required for effective interprofessional working', in G. Barret, D. Sellman and J. Thomas (eds) *Interprofessional working in health and social care: Professional perspectives*, Basingstoke: Palgrave, pp 18-31.

Barret, G., Greenwood, R. and Ross, K. (2003) 'Integrating interprofessional education into 10 health and social care programmes', *Journal of Interprofessional Care*, vol 17, no 3, pp 293-301.

Bateman, H., Bailey, P. and McLellan, H. (2003) 'Of rocks and safe channels: learning to navigate as an interprofessional team', *Journal of Interprofessional Care*, vol 17, no 2, pp 141-50.

Beck, U. and Beck-Gernsheim, E. (2002) *Individualisation: Institutionalised individualism and its social and political consequences*, London: Sage Publications.

Blättel-Mink, B. and Kuhlmann, E. (2003) 'Health professions, gender and society: introduction and outlook', *International Journal of Sociology and Social Policy*, vol 23, no 4/5, pp 1-21.

Bourgeault, I.L., Benoit, C. and Davies-Floyd, R. (eds) (2004) *Reconceiving midwifery*, Kingston/Montreal: McGill-Queen's University Press.

Broadbent, J. (1998) 'Practice nurses and effects on the new general practitioner contract in the British NHS: the advent of a professional project?', *Social Science and Medicine*, vol 47, pp 497-506.

D'Amour, D., Ferrada-Videla, M., San Martin Rodriguez, L. and Beaulieu, M.D. (2005) 'Conceptual basis for interprofessional collaboration: core concepts and theoretical frameworks', *Journal of Interprofessional Care*, vol 19 (suppl 1), pp 116-31.

Davies, C. (2000) 'Getting health professionals to work together', *British Medical Journal*, vol 320, pp 1021-2.

Delhey, J. and Newton, K. (2003) 'Who trusts? The origins of social trust in seven societies', *European Societies*, vol 5, no 2, pp 93-138.

Dingwall, R., Rafferty, A.M. and Webster, C. (1991) *An introduction to the social history of nursing*, London: Routledge.

Domajnko, B., Kvas, A., Štrancar, K., Bojc, N. and Pahor, M. (2006) 'Živeta interprofesionalna razmerja: kvalitativni pogled', in A. Kvas, M. Pahor, D. Klemenc and J. Šmitek (eds) *Sodelovanje med medicinskimi sestrami in zdravniki v zdravstvenem timu: Priložnost za izboljševanje kakovosti*, Ljubljana: DMSBZT Ljubljana, pp 235-59.

Essex, C. (1995) 'Nursing eulogies ignored ethos of control and punishment', *British Medical Journal*, vol 311, p 873.

Freidson, E. (1994) *Professionalism reborn: Theory, prophecy and policy*, Cambridge: Polity Press.

Hean, S., Macleod Clarke, J., Adams, K., Humphris, D. and Lathlean, J. (2006) 'Being seen by others as we see ourselves: the congruence between ingroup and outgroup perceptions of health and social care students', *Learning in Health and Social Care*, vol 5, no 1, pp 10-22.

Hojat, M., Gonella, J.S., Nasca, T.J., Fields, S.K., Cicchetti, A., Lo Scalzo, A., Taroni, F., Amicosante, A.M.V., Macinati, M., Tangucci, M., Liva, C., Ricciardi, G., Eidelman, S., Admi, H., Geva, H., Mashiach, T., Alroy, G., Alcorta-Gonzales, A., Ibarra, D. and Torres-Ruiz, A. (2003) 'Comparisons of American, Israeli, Italian and Mexican physicians and nurses on the total and factor scores of the Jefferson scale of attitudes towards physician–nurse collaborative relationships', *International Journal of Nursing Studies*, vol 40, no 4, pp 427-35.

Iglič, H. (2004) 'Dejavniki nizke stopnje zaupanja v Sloveniji', *Družboslovne razprave*, vol XX, no 46/47, pp 149-75.

Inglehart, R. (1997) *Modernization and postmodernization: Cultural, economic and political change in 43 societies*, Princeton, NJ: Princeton University Press.

Inglehart, R. (1999) 'Trust, well-being and democracy', in M.E. Warren (ed) *Democracy and trust*, Cambridge: Cambridge University Press, pp 88-120.

Klemenc, D. and Pahor, M. (eds) (2001) *Medicinske sestre v Sloveniji*, Ljubljana: Društvo MS in ZT Ljubljana.

Klemenc, D., Kvas, A., Pahor, M. and Smitek, J. (eds) (2003) *Zdravstvena nega v luči etike*, Ljubljana: Društvo MS in ZT Ljubljana.

Kollock, P. (1998) 'Social dilemmas: the anatomy of cooperation', *Annual Review of Sociology*, vol 24, pp 183-214.

Lempp, H. and Seale, C. (2004) 'The hidden curriculum in undergraduate medical education: qualitative study of medical students' perceptions of teaching', *British Medical Journal*, vol 329, pp 770-3.

Mickan, S.M. and Rodgers, S.A. (2005) 'Effective health care teams: a model of six characteristics developed from shared perceptions', *Journal of Interprofessional Care*, vol 19, no 4, pp 358-70.

Pethybridge, J. (2004) 'How team working influence discharge planning from hospital: a study of four multidisciplinary teams in an acute hospital in England', *Journal of Interprofessional Care*, vol 18, no 1, pp 29-41.

Pollard, K., Miers, M. and Gilchrist, M. (2004) 'Collaborative learning for collaborative working? Initial findings from a longitudinal study of health and social care students', *Health and Social Care in the Community*, vol 12, no 4, pp 346-58.

Rafferty, A.M., Ball, J. and Aiken, L.H. (2001) 'Are teamwork and professional autonomy compatible, and do they result in improved hospital care?', *Quality in Health Care*, vol 10 (suppl II), pp 32-7.

Ryan, A.A. (1996) 'Doctor–nurse relations: a review of the literature', *Social Science in Health: International Journal of Research and Practice*, vol 2, no 2, pp 93-106.

Saks, M. and Kuhlmann, E. (2006) 'Introduction: professions, social inclusion and citizenship: challenge and change in European health systems', *Knowledge, Work and Society*, vol 4, no 1, pp 9-20.

Salvage, J. and Smith, R. (2000) 'Doctors and nurses: doing it differently', *British Medical Journal*, vol 320, pp 1019-20.

San Martin Rodriguez, L., Beaulieu, M.D., D'Amour, D. and Ferrada-Videla, M. (2005) 'The determinants of successful collaboration: a review of theoretical and empirical work', *Journal of Interprofessional Care*, vol 19 (suppl 1), pp 132-47.

Skela-Savič, B., Pagon, M. and Lobnikar, B. (2006) 'Organizacijska kultura v slovenskih bolnišnicah', in V. Rajkovic (ed) *Management sprememb: Zbornik 25. Mednarodne konference o razvoju organizacijskih znanosti*, Proceedings of the 25th International Conference on Organizational Science Development, Slovenia, Portorož, March, Kranj: Moderna organizacija, pp 1145-53.

Soederberg, A. (1999) 'The practical wisdom of enrolled nurses, registered nurses and physicians in situation of ethical difficulty in intensive care', PhD thesis, Umea, Umea University Medical Faculty.

Strauss, A.L. (1995) *Qualitative analysis for social scientists*, Cambridge: Cambridge University Press.

Thomas, E.J., Sexton, J.B. and Helmreich, R.L. (2003) 'Discrepant attitudes about teamwork among critical care nurses and physicians', *Critical Care Medicine*, vol 31, no 3, pp 956-9.

Toš, N. (ed) (2004) *Vrednote v prehodu III: Slovensko javno mnenje 1999-2004*, Ljubljana: Fakulteta za družbene vede, IDV CJMMK.

Walby, S. and Greenwell, J. (1994) *Medicine and nursing*, London: Sage Publications.

Wensing, M., Wollersheim, H. and Grol, R. (2006) 'Organizational interventions to implement improvements in patient care: a structured review of reviews', *Implementation Science*, vol 1, no 2, doi:10.1186/1748-5908-I-2, www.implementationscience.com/content/I/I/2

Witz, A. and Annandale, E. (2006) 'The challenge of nursing', in D. Kelleher, J. Gabe and G. Williams (eds) *Challenging medicine* (2nd edition), London: Routledge, pp 24-39.

Zwarenstein, M. and Bryant, W. (2004) *Interventions to promote collaboration between nurses and doctors*, The Cochrane Library, vol 3, http://gateway.ut.ovid.com/gw1/ovidweb.cgi

Educating generalists: flexibility and identity in auxiliary nursing in Finland[1]

Sirpa Wrede

Introduction

The discourse of professionalism, consisting of a set of normative values and identities, is currently spreading to new occupational and organisational contexts (Evetts, 2003). It is a mechanism for the control of work and workers, mobilised by employers as a form of self-discipline for employees (Fournier, 1999). The discourse of professionalism is employed in organisations as an ideology of occupational powers to divide work within and between occupations (Fournier, 2000). This chapter examines the dynamics of this discourse in the context of changes in the welfare state, taking both its disciplinary and enabling aspects into account. The constitution of a normative professional identity is considered a collective achievement that builds on the internal and external claims made. In turn, the normative professional identity that the discourse of professionalism offers as a point of reference plays a vital role in the way individual professionals make sense of their workplace reality. The analysis thus links the shaping of micro-level experiences to macro-level actions.

The flexibilisation of Finnish auxiliary nursing started with the educational reform that was introduced in the early 1990s. It included the training of healthcare assistants, social service assistants, paramedics, childcare workers and similar occupations. The central aim in combining a health and social care orientation in one occupation was to make it more flexible from the point of view of service management. As a result, the paths leading to the new degree and the actual skills acquired through education vary greatly. The creation of the new practical nurse as an official occupational category is an example of public policy support for organisational professionalism. This chapter examines how the discourse of flexibility is reflected in the professional identities of workers in this new occupational class.

So-called 'support workers' in professional services are of central theoretical interest for the study of the dynamics of professional fields (see also Saks, this volume). In the traditional taxonomic approach to the study of professions, auxiliary nursing, when recognised at all, is conceptualised as a 'non-profession' and demoted by the terminology 'auxiliaries' or 'support workers'. Such confining terminology carries organisational discourse about divisions of labour in healthcare. Although their occupational titles underscore their subordinate position, professionals belonging to these groups are often expected to carry out complex work independently (Stacey, 1984). The discursive separations in healthcare successfully separate medicine from the mundane task of 'caring', traditionally viewed as an essentially female activity. The masculine science of 'curing', on the other hand, is construed as essentially different and the most important activity in healthcare organisations (Davies, 1992). Furthermore, analytical attention to the divisions within caring has remained scarce, even though the academisation of nursing has further deepened such divisions. When research focuses on the powerful groups, it indirectly validates the claims of these groups.

An alternative is offered by the new sociology of professional groups in which the focus has shifted from a preoccupation with defining 'profession' to analysis of the appeal of professionalism (Evetts, 2003). Instead of understanding occupational change as a result of separate professional projects, it is useful to conceptualise it in the wider context of professional fields (Fournier, 2000). Changes in occupations thus cannot be construed without the work system that enfolds them. In order to understand how professional power is discursively achieved, research needs to examine how actual practices seek to legitimise hierarchy. A closer look at the mundane activities that constitute the cultural life-worlds of the different healthcare actors is perceived as a fruitful approach to understanding power relations in healthcare.

This chapter examines the flexibilisation of Finnish auxiliary nursing, providing an example of the effects of policy changes on the workforce and highlighting the highly complex nature of workforce change. The qualitative analysis is based on policy documents and on a set of 15 thematic interviews with recently graduated practical nurses working in care for the elderly. Starting with an outline of the analytical approach, the chapter then presents empirical findings on the impact of policy changes on the shaping of Finnish auxiliary nursing. This is followed by findings from the interview data, focusing on how occupational identity and concepts of professionalism take shape at the micro level. The final section presents conclusions about the relationship between organisational discourse of flexibility and professionalism. The argument is that, even though Finnish care workers still take pride in their work and in their professional identity, flexibilisation hinders the development of collective notions of occupational professionalism. Instead, professional identities are fragmented and when engagement occurs, it concerns the workplace rather than the occupation.

Power resources and the dynamics of professionalism

For the professional workforce providing public services, social policy constitutes the major influence shaping its social and cultural composition. From the 1930s onwards, the state-centred welfare regimes that emerged in the UK and in the Nordic countries supported and demanded a professional ethos that T.M. Marshall (1939) envisioned as social service professionalism. Specific to the Nordic countries is that state-centred welfare regimes built universalistic 'servicing states' to cater for social care needs to a greater extent than other welfare regimes (Esping-Andersen, 1999). The universalistic Finnish welfare state created social care services, like day care for children, and care for the elderly and disabled people, that even the middle classes came to rely on (Anttonen and Sipilä, 1996).

Currently, however, trends shaping public care in Finland exemplify what has been called an attack on social service professionalism (Hanlon, 1998) or an attack on the ethics of caring (Julkunen, 1991). The neoliberal critique of the welfare state is typically argued in economic terms. Its discourse has a material base in the politics of retrenchment and effectiveness. Accordingly, universalistic welfare states – former welfare state 'leaders' – are under neoliberal attack and cast as 'laggards' in economic growth (Korpi, 2001). In Finland as elsewhere, reformers target social service professionalism as an ineffective and costly way to organise professional services. The neoliberal critique portrays the professional groups that provide social services as inflexible protectors of their turfs (Julkunen, 1991). Apart from seeking to make service production more flexible and effective, the neoliberal reforms of the Finnish public sector are associated with privatisation, particularly of many aspects of social care, and the dismantling of the centralised steering and planning system (Julkunen, 2001). Reflecting this critique, redirected social policy aims to encourage trans-sectoral collaboration and the creation of multiprofessional teams.

Such 'population responsibility' programmes are reminiscent of community care reforms in the UK where the emerging market for professional services demands a new, commercialised version of professionalism that some professions (or elements of professions) encounter and internalise, and thus become 'winners' (Hanlon, 1997). However, there are also 'losers' in the new professional fields. Hanlon (1998) identifies fragmentation of previously relatively homogeneous professions and the struggle of professional groups to legitimise working practices.

Theorising transitions in the discourse of professionalism

What are the determinants of this win–or–lose process in the changing context of the welfare state? The starting point here is that different occupational groups in care work have different access to the means to initiate professional projects. I adopt a discursive-materialist perspective: in order to be effective and powerful, a discourse needs a material base in established social institutions and practices (Weedon, 1987). Discursive practices are embedded in material power relations, which need to be transformed before change can happen. The recognition of materiality of power leads me to apply power resources theory, a familiar approach in state theory (see, for instance, Korpi, 1998). This approach enables us to conceptualise the 'labour of divisions' in a professional field, which Fournier (2000) identifies as a distributive process. At the core is the production and distribution of professional chances among workers, whose interests are unequally represented. Power resources theory has been extensively used to analyse levels and changes of industrial conflict in Western nations. A key argument is that the probability of open conflict diminishes between actors with great power disparities; instead, actors (managers of power resources) move potentially costly distributive processes to institutions (Korpi, 1985). This offers a promising alternative to the perspective of professional struggles dogged by open conflict.

From the point of view of distributive processes in professional fields the state emerges as the arena where professional groups are able to institutionalise their resources through formal recognition of the service they provide. Roberts and Dietrich (1999) identify two independent dynamics of professional organisation. The first, the sociological rationale, is related to the degree of social recognition for the service the group provides and also to the occupation's ability to organise its power resources effectively in society, that is, to engage in making claims as a recognised interest group. The second, the economic rationale, is based on the economic exchanges related to professional services. In the economic literature that focuses on market conditions, a profession is conceptualised as a strategic network made up of separately operating but interdependent practitioners whose aim is to maintain and develop core competencies that help practitioners lower transaction costs associated with earning rent for the exchange of knowledge (Savage, 1994). Knowledge is thus the strategic resource on which professional networks capitalise. Under non-free market conditions, where a profession controls the application of professional knowledge, professions are therefore necessary institutions in the economic sense (Roberts and Dietrich, 1999). Managed care reforms in the US are a prime example of how loss of control over such core competencies impinges on the authority and autonomy of even the strong professions, as it weakens the economic rationale for their professional status (Savage and Robertson, 1997).

Paradoxically, the flexiblisation of Finnish auxiliary nursing offers a similar example, even though its 'professionalisation' is of recent date. For a long time, the example considered here – public elderly care – was perceived as a replacement for women's traditional, private-sphere, non-skilled care work. In the 1980s, a humanitarian, holistic view of care centred round individual needs occurring in the natural ageing process became the starting point for social policy (Paasivaara, 2002). From this social-gerontological perspective, home care was recast as social care with the charter to support the client in everyday life situations, allowing them to continue to live at home as long as possible with assistance that took their individual lifestyle into account (Tedre, 1999). Since the 1990s, neoliberal reformers have sought to shift the emphasis from residential to home care, but the impetus for reform has come from its supposed economic efficiency. Proponents of the humanitarian approach supported the shift, hoping for more holistic care. Expectations of greater individuality in care, however, have largely been betrayed. The core of municipal policies has been to make home care more effective and to curtail public responsibility for elderly care, both in terms of scope and coverage.

In practice, home care is now limited to the medical and physical needs of the client. The preparation of meals, shopping for groceries and cleaning are organised separately and provided by other than public providers. From the point of view of care receivers, the medicalisation of care thus parallels the fragmentation of services. The new form of auxiliary nursing is the key policy instrument to revive home care for the elderly. On the surface, the emphasis on this flexible workforce constitutes an 'upgrading' of home care, as home helps with no formal qualifications give way to practical nurses. The explanation of this increased reliance on credentials is that the medicalised service depends on a workforce that can also carry out nursing tasks, albeit within the narrow confines of practical nursing. In reality, autonomy is lost, as care at the home is organised in a Taylorist fashion, not holistically as before (Wrede and Henriksson, 2005).

An analysis of the managerialist organisational discourse demonstrates that a set of values lies at its core, which contributes to an ideology of 'flexible professionalism' (see also Dahle and Skogheim, this volume). The proper professional conduct of practical nurses is linked with the ability to work flexibly in different types of work roles and across sectors, depending on the needs of the employers. Flexibilisation is a parallel process of, and linked to, the commercialisation of professionalism (Hanlon, 1997, 1998; Fournier, 2000). The discourse of flexibility gives rise to a discipline that structures the work of professional groups that lack resources to defend their work roles in workplaces.

The analytical approach

The government of the occupations can be conceptualised as a process of formulating organisational charters and missions, as well as professional licences and mandates (Dingwall and Strong, 1997; Wrede, 2001). These concepts can be used to analytically separate organisational and occupational professionalism. Organisational charters and professional licences are instruments employed from above to shape professionalism. By contrast, claim making that arises within a group – as part of occupational professionalism – is based on the tactic of collective action. If occupations are studied within interacting systems and not individually, it is evident that no one group has hegemonic power over the shaping of organisational missions and the issue of material and discursive power resources emerges as a vital focus for research.

The flexibilisation of practical nursing in institutions and policy

Since the 1940s, the Finnish healthcare system has relied on a trained lower-level nurse workforce. The first auxiliary nurses were trained for practical bedside care, particularly for the care of patients with chronic illnesses. As social services expanded, other groups of carers with similar social and educational profiles were created for both health and social care, each with their own curriculum and educational institution. Until the late 1970s, the policy considered auxiliary nurses simply as 'nursing assistants'. However, the universalistic welfare state began to assign new roles and promoted these groups with two particular measures. First, policies invested in increasing their social recognition. For example, in the early 1980s auxiliary nursing was recast as 'primary nursing', with a defined area of expertise. 'Primary nurses' worked in large numbers both in residential care facilities for the elderly and in hospitals providing acute medical care. The economic foundation for 'primary nursing' arose from the expansion of the Finnish public sector during this period when there was a shortage of nurses. The reform extended their training curriculum from one and a half to two and a half years.

The development of social services was central to the universalistic welfare state, reflecting its overall emphasis on social citizenship rights. The expansion of services presupposed not only a workforce that was larger, but also qualitatively renewed; educational policy thus became a central instrument of social policy. The work of occupations such as 'primary nurses' and social carers became linked to a knowledge base, even though the control of that knowledge was in the hands of expert civil servants (Tedre, 1999; Paasivaara, 2002). They were 'social planners', a new profession within the welfare state bureaucracy. They drafted an organisational charter, for instance, for municipal home making and home help, defining it as social care for families with children and for the elderly. In everyday work, the practical knowledge and values associated with traditional womanhood merged with the holistic social agenda of the new home care (Tedre, 1999). The organisational discourse of the universalistic welfare state can be interpreted as an enabling framework that elevated both the position of care receivers and that of care givers.

Egalitarianism was at the core of the Nordic welfare regimes of the universalistic type during their 'mature state' in the 1970s and 1980s (Esping-Andersen, 1999). This ideology gave rise to policies aimed at equal opportunities in education, equality between men and women and equality in the workplace. The goal was to weed out the elitist practices of old professional groups, for instance by removing outer signs of occupational hierarchy. The discourse contributed to a flattening of professional hierarchies, although cultural and social changes took longer to occur than swings in political discourse. Nevertheless, egalitarianism provided a rationale for extending social recognition to lower-level groups whose work had hitherto gained very little appreciation.

The second route to occupational change in the universalistic welfare state concerns the improved economic position of the lower-level carers in its institutional framework. For instance, in the primary health centres created in the 1970s, all personnel groups were salaried full-time employees (Wrede, 2001). The management of hospitals also reflected the new 'equalitarian' ideas about work organisation, even though these institutions were more resistant to change than the new primary health centres (Eriksson-Piela, 2003). The most important economic basis for the improved professional opportunities of lower-level carers was the general introduction of economics into care in the family (Anttonen and

Sipilä, 1996; Esping-Andersen, 1999). In addition to providing social services to others, carers themselves also benefited from the existence of universal access to social services (Henriksson et al, 2006).

When the politics of the welfare state took a new course in the 1990s, the shift contributed to the rise of a new type of organisational discourse concerning lower-level carers. The current form of Finnish certification for regulated carers and auxiliaries was introduced in 1993 on the basis of a new joint curriculum for health and social care, replacing seven earlier occupations in healthcare and three in social care. The new occupational title *lähihoitaja* emphasises the idea of the carer being close to the client. The aim of the curriculum for practical nurses was to create versatile and flexible carers. Legislation only protects their occupational title, the tasks they do in workplaces can generally also be done by non-trained workers. The secondary-level education for practical nurses was initially two and a half years, of which the last six months were spent studying one of the several alternative orientations. However, the emphasis was on providing general competence (Rintala and Elovainio, 1997). In 1999, in response to criticism, training was extended to three years, one of which is devoted to a specialisation study programme. The same year, the decision was taken to apply skills tests in vocational education in order to assess students' competence and to evaluate training. In the training for practical nurses, skills tests were implemented in 2006, providing employers' representatives greater influence than before (Finnish National Board of Education, 2005). The multiple routes leading to a certified practical nurse degree include a competence-based qualification, apprenticeship and applied programmes for specific groups such as the unemployed or migrants (Ministry of Health and Social Affairs, 2001). This was considered necessary to meet a future shortfall. It is calculated that more than 10% of each cohort of the Finnish youth need to be brought in to the occupation, although growing numbers of more mature students are also being recruited (Vuorensyrjä et al, 2006).

The discourse of education policy defines the practical nurses as a flexible workforce that can be assigned to basic care and nursing tasks. The goals of education policy complement and sometimes compete with those of social policy. In neoliberal social policy, practical nurses are seen as the flexible workforce that is particularly needed for routine, work-intensive care domains that lie on the borderline between healthcare and social care.

Occupational identity and professionalism in the workplace

At first glance, the educational discourse of the versatile and flexible practical nurse promotes care workers. However, its effects in the workplace have turned out to be disempowering. This is related to the differences in the material bases of this discourse compared to earlier discourse. Whereas the universal welfare state invested in expanding the workforce and in giving that workforce secure terms of employment, the flexibility discourse has served the needs of employers at a time when resources from welfare services have been cut. The shrinking resources spent on elderly care, for instance, have structured the lives of professionals concretely, as temporary contracts have become common. Additionally, the informants in the present study report understaffing as a regular occurrence. Many cite lack of time for adequate care as a chronic feature of elderly care. They describe their encounter with what has been identified by Davies (1992) in a study of British nursing as 'coping management', practised by the managers of relatively powerless groups in a professional field, as a response to inadequate resources. This inward management style – which in the end reinforces organisational neglect – is hard on the subordinates, as it overstretches their capacity and creates an environment that is not supportive or caring of individual members of the staff (Davies, 1992).

In the following account, I analyse practical nurses' experiences. A constant theme in the accounts of practical nurses is how their superiors in the workplace automatically assign them to the status of subordinates. My argument is that their lack of professional authority is produced in the workplace interactions through discursive and cultural practices that have links to other levels of organisational discourse.

Unclear boundaries: being a 'Jane-of-all-trades'

From the point of view of practical nurses, coping management has two key components. First, the ideal of versatility translates into the expectation that a nurse should be a 'Jane-of-all-trades'. The 15 informants in the present study work in different types of institutional settings, including home care, different types of residential care or combinations of the two. Despite this diversity, they describe their work roles in very similar terms: what they are and are not 'allowed' to do. Practical nurses often experience a lack of trust in their abilities in the workplace on the part of other professionals, as they are perceived as capable of doing 'a bit of everything but not quite anything' (H6), as one participant in the study put it. The blurred boundaries of their work role are also reflected in the tasks that the carers are asked to do that they do not feel are their 'proper' tasks, such as preparing meals for residents in a service housing facility.

The informants identified the scope of their work roles with the work setting rather than with education:

> '[What you are able to do] is dependent on the place, for example this distribution of medication. It was so thoroughly taught in the school, how to calculate medication and other such things. In the first place where I worked, we were allowed to distribute the drugs. In this place we have no business at the medicine cabinet. So it should not have been so important in the training.' (H10)

The same informant noted that vagueness had already existed in the training programme: 'The responsibility was on the places where we had our practical training, [they decided] how active they were to teach' (H10).

Practical nurses often cited 'house rules' as a framework that structures and defines the work of a practical nurse. From their perspective, house rules appear definite and impersonal, leaving little or no room for the discretion of the carer. When practical nurses reflect on their working conditions, the majority classifies work contexts simply as good or bad, often with reference to the house rules and the way these apply to them in practice. Their experience reflects the resourcing of services, often characterised by organisational neglect and related coping management. Some institutions for the long-term care of frail elderly people have an infamous reputation among carers, specifically because of the effects they have on carers themselves. In their eyes, the overstretching of the staff turns carers into robots, and one of their worst fears is that they will become one. They said 'just wait a few years and you'll be the same' (H1). Several of the informants declared that they were prepared to make compromises in order to work somewhere where they felt the workplace supported them, where 'one is allowed to show one's skills, to do what one is able to do' (H5).

Women's work: subordination and lack of power

The second feature of coping management concerns the experience of being subjected to practices of subordination. This was described by one of the informants as being made into a 'dish rag'. The widespread lack of trust in the abilities of practical nurses leads to efforts to narrow down the scope of their practice. The dish rag treatment involves denial of a work role that includes rewarding, clean and light tasks. Instead it is limited to tasks that are dirty, heavy and unrewarding: '[Others] say that's not caring, or yes, it is caring but not [the practical nurse's] task, that [she] should be cleaning the toilet' (H2). The dish rag treatment is disempowering. Practical nurses often portray themselves as subordinate workers, who lack the resources of stronger groups in the labour market: 'In this kind of women-dominated branch you can't easily go on strike, I don't think that could happen [in elderly care]' (H5).

Practical nurses further describe organisational practices that teach them the boundaries of their practice. At least from their perspective, this separates them from nurses and doctors, who, they assume, possess unquestionable competence. A central practice involves requiring practical nurses to give proof of even the simplest nursing tasks that have been included in their training:

> 'First we take our training, then we still have to give proof [of the ability to distribute medication] when we start working, in every new workplace, and every six months. No other professional group whose training qualifies them to distribute medication needs to give proofs after school. Apparently there are some things that influence this, like some doctor's name, signature in the paper, as if the doctor would have seen me distributing the medication, even less that I have given someone an injection.' (H11)

As the practice of giving proofs varies between workplaces and even within the same workplace – and as it is often seen as a mere red tape procedure that lacks real relevance – practical nurses often feel they are subjected to arbitrary organisational power. Some go as far as to question these limitations, but they are seldom in a position to actively challenge these.

The other side of the flexibility discourse concerns unreasonable expectations of skill in the organisation. At a time when practical nurses are prepared to take on more responsibility for the tasks they trained for, they resent being assigned unclear responsibilities for tasks, such as the duty to monitor the side-effects of medication on elderly clients, for which they share responsibility with doctors or nurses. This situation is made more complicated by their subordinate professional position. One informant complained: 'even if you asked a doctor to go through that medication file and check if there is something that could be taken away, they seldom do' (H5). The lack of resources forces carers sometimes to prioritise even the basic needs of the care receivers. Clients and their relatives sometimes interpret organisational neglect as neglect on the part of individual carers: '[The relatives] say the carers do things no one should do; ... they don't understand that [when] we don't have enough personnel, we can't manage' (H12).

Informants mention the marginal position of their work in society more often than its gendered character. Feelings of disempowerment colour their accounts. When asked about the most suitable sort of person for this occupation, or when reflecting on their own choice to enter the training, several of our informants described it as a last resort occupation. Becoming a practical nurse was associated with previous exclusions, due to a lack of engagement in studies or lack of success in the labour market.

Flexibility and professionalism

This chapter has discussed professionalism from a discursive perspective and identified the material bases of discourses. The process identified here is a shift in the organisational discourse of the Finnish welfare state from egalitarian social service professionalism to flexible professionalism.

In the post-war era some countries, including Finland, succeeded in redirecting many distributive conflicts from the labour market into democratic politics. During the 1970s and the 1980s, when gender relations in Finnish society were under renegotiation, the same means were used to solve the rising conflicts between women's paid work and their unpaid care work. In comparative terms, the Nordic servicing state heavily relied on low-status care occupations precisely to respond to such new care needs (Esping-Andersen, 1999). The elevation of this status was one aspect of the so-called woman-friendly welfare state. In Finland developments since the 1990s have resulted in the redirection and narrowing down of the servicing state. The call for flexibility as a basis for organising auxiliary nursing is an example of how the change of direction in welfare policy is achieved in practice. This chapter has examined the discursive formulation of flexibility and the ways it is put into practice both at macro and micro levels. The analysis points to contradictions in the discourse; the egalitarian rhetoric of the universalistic era continues to be employed in education. However, the pervasive, fundamental feature of the flexibility discourse on the education of practical nurses is the dissolution of their occupational boundaries, reflecting the demands of employers for effectiveness.

The flexibility discourse re-establishes the workplace as the central arena for the shaping of the occupation of auxiliary nursing. In this context, this chapter identifies an inward-oriented management style that is rooted in responding to organisational neglect with coping strategies rather than tackling the lack of resources. Practical nurses, who are expected to be versatile and subordinate simultaneously, balance between their unstable work roles and the often unreasonable expectations they encounter in workplace interactions. Practical nurses' failure to meet the expectations placed on them results in disappointments for clients and colleagues and in discontent for themselves. They also identify an institutionalised distrust, as expressed in the practice of proof giving, which undermines the relevance of the credentials they have acquired through training.

Practical nurses often feel disempowered in the workplace, as they are 'treated like someone's dish rag'. Work organisation limits their work role to only include the heavy aspects of work that are to be carried out at a forced pace. Neoliberal reforms have thus helped to reinstitutionalise distrust and disempowerment that lower-level carers encounter in their everyday workplace interactions. Consequently, the organisational rhetoric of versatility and empowerment of the practical nurses as the 'closest carers' nurtures disempowerment, as, in one way or another, they constantly fall short of providing what is expected of them. Their disempowerment stretches beyond the workplace. Society's low appreciation of care work is reflected in organisational neglect – and this is disempowering. Practical nurses see themselves through the eyes of society as second-class workers, who do work that others, more fortunate or more talented people, can avoid.

The analysis bears witness to the tenaciousness and vitality of gendered power resources in professional fields (Bourgeault, 2005; Henriksson et al, 2006). Neoliberal reforms have returned important aspects of social care to the private sphere, either to be dealt with through informal care or through services bought in the market. At the same time, healthcare largely remains a public responsibility. The traditional division of caring and curing thus reappears in a modernised version. This chapter shows how the discourse of flexibility reinforces this division. The medico-managerial culture of the new elderly care in Finland assigns practical nurses the position as flexible workers under house rules. As the social needs of clients are reconceptualised as the responsibility of the 'family', there no longer exists an *economic* rationale for the state to promote professionalisation of social care.

In the feminist debates of the 1980s, the Nordic welfare state was praised for being woman-friendly just because it shared the reproductive responsibilities that previously had been women's informal work. Even though care remained women's work, its institutional framework recognised its economic and social value. The neoliberal flexibilisation discourse denies both economic rationale and social recognition for the occupational professionalism of social care occupations. In the building of the flexibility discourse, the policy makers are able to make use of both the gendered expectations that still are in place for women to be caring and the traditional values associated with professionalism to view their work as a vocation. This is reflected in the efforts of practical nurses to hold on to their dignity as carers. Even under pressure they resist 'turning into robots'. Thus, flexibility is a disciplinary discourse in the Foucauldian sense of self-governance that supports a normative professional identity which presupposes individualised subordinance to coping management rather than collective resistance to organisational neglect.

Note

[1] The work reported in this chapter was funded through the Academy of Finland project 'New Dynamics of Professionalism within Caring Occupations' (#211270). The interviews were conducted by Malin Grönholm, Laura Tainio and myself in spring 2004 using an interview guide developed in collaboration with Lea Henriksson and her research project 'The Politics of Recruitment'.

References

Anttonen, A. and Sipilä, J. (1996) 'European social care services: is it possible to identify models?', *Journal of European Social Policy*, vol 6, no 2, pp 87-100.

Bourgeault, I.L. (2005) 'Rationalization of health care and female professional projects', *Knowledge, Work and Society*, vol 3, no 1, pp 25-52.

Davies, C. (1992) 'Gender, history and management style in nursing: towards a theoretical synthesis', in M. Savage and A. Witz (eds) *Gender and bureaucracy*, Oxford: Blackwell, pp 229-52.

Dingwall, R. and Strong, P. (1997) 'The interactional study of organizations: a critique and reformulation', in G. Miller and R. Dingwall (eds) *Context and method in qualitative research*, London: Sage Publications, pp 139-54.

Eriksson-Piela, S. (2003) *Tunnetta, tietoa vai hierarkiaa? Sairaanhoidon moninainen ammatillisuus*, Tampere: University of Tampere.

Esping-Andersen, G. (1999) *Social foundations of postindustrial economics*, Oxford: Oxford University Press.

Evetts, J. (2003) 'The sociological analysis of professionalism: occupational change in the modern world', *International Sociology*, vol 18, pp 395-415.

Finnish National Board of Education (2005) *The implications of using skills tests as a basis for a National Evaluation System in Finland*, Helsinki: Finnish National Board of Education.

Fournier, V. (1999) 'The appeal to "professionalism" as a disciplinary mechanism', *The Sociological Review*, vol 47, no 2, pp 280-307.

Fournier, V. (2000) 'Boundary work and the (un)making of the professions', in N. Malin (ed) *Professionalism, boundaries and the workplace*, London: Routledge, pp 67–86.

Hanlon, G. (1997) 'A profession in transition? Lawyers, the market and significant others', *The Modern Law Review*, vol 60, no 6, pp 798–822.

Hanlon, G. (1998) 'Professionalism as enterprise: service class politics and the redefinition of professionalism', *Sociology*, vol 32, pp 43–63.

Henriksson, L., Wrede, S. and Burau, V. (2006) 'Understanding professional projects in welfare service work: revival of old professionalism?', *Gender, Work & Organization*, vol 13, no 2, pp 174–92.

Julkunen, R. (1991) 'Hoiva ja professionalismi', *Sosiologia*, vol 28, no 2, pp 75–83.

Julkunen, R. (2001) *Suunnanmuutos: 1990-luvun sosiaalipoliittinen reformi Suomessa*, Tampere: Vastapaino.

Korpi, W. (1985) 'Power resources approach vs. action and conflict: on causal and intentional explanations in the study of power', *Sociological Theory*, vol 3, no 2, pp 31–45.

Korpi, W. (1998) 'The iceberg of power below the surface: a preface to power resources theory', in J. O'Connor and G. Olsen (eds) *Power resources theory and the welfare state*, Toronto: University of Toronto Press, pp xi–xiv.

Korpi, W. (2001) 'The economic consequences of Sweden's welfare state: does the causal analysis hold?', *Challenge*, November–December (retrieved through LookSmart, 22 March 2006).

Marshall, T.M. (1939) 'The recent history of professionalism in relation to social structure and social policy', *The Canadian Journal of Economics and Political Science*, vol 5, no 3, pp 325–40.

Ministry of Health and Social Affairs (2001) *Sosiaali- ja terveydenhuollon ennakointityöryhmän mietintö*, Committee report 2001:7, Helsinki: Ministry of Health and Social Affairs.

Paasivaara, L. (2002) *Suomalaisen vanhusten hoitotyön muotoutuminen monitasotarkastelussa 1930-luvulta 2000-luvulle*, Oulu: University of Oulu.

Rintala, T. and Elovainio, M. (1997) *Lähihoitajien työ, ammatti-identiteetti ja hyvinvointi*, Helsinki: Stakes.

Roberts, J. and Dietrich, M. (1999) 'Conceptualizing professionalism: why economics needs sociology', *American Journal of Economics and Sociology*, vol 58, no 4, pp 977–98.

Savage, D.A. (1994) 'The professions in theory and history: the case of pharmacy', *Business and Economic History*, vol 23, no 2, pp 129–60.

Savage, D.A. and Robertson, P. (1997) 'The maintenance of professional authority: the case of physicians and hospitals in the United States', in P. Robertson (ed) *Authority and control in modern industry*, London: Routledge, pp 155–72.

Stacey, M. (1984) 'Who are the health workers? Patients and other unpaid workers in health care', *Economic and Industrial Democracy*, vol 5, no 10, pp 157–84.

Tedre, S. (1999) *Hoivan sanattomat sopimukset: Tutkimus vanhusten kotipalvelun työntekijöiden työstä*, Joensuu: University of Joensuu.

Vuorensyrjä, M., Borgman, M., Kemppainen, T., Mäntysaari, M. and Pohjola, A. (2006) *Sosiaalialan osaajat*, Jyväskylä: Jyväskylän yliopisto.

Weedon, C. (1987) *Feminist practice and poststructuralist theory*, Oxford: Blackwell.

Wrede, S. (2001) *Decentering care for mothers: The politics of midwifery and the design of Finnish maternity services*, Turku: Åbo Akademi University Press.

Wrede, S. and Henriksson, L. (2005) 'The changing terms of welfare service work: Finnish home care in transition', in H.M. Dahl and T.R. Eriksen (eds) *Dilemmas of care in the Nordic welfare state: Continuity and change*, Aldershot: Ashgate, pp 62–79.

NINE

Culture matters: integration of folk medicine into healthcare in Russia[1]

Elena Iarskaia-Smirnova and Pavel Romanov

Introduction

The integration of complementary and alternative medicine (CAM) into orthodox healthcare systems and the professionalisation of these services are global phenomena. These developments place new challenges on both the governance of healthcare and the dominance of orthodox medicine (Saks, 2006). However, national governments and professional bodies respond in different ways to these new demands. Integration and professionalisation are driven by various forces and the success of new professional projects is uneven. This chapter explores the processes of integration of CAM into the official healthcare system in Russia. It places the demand for, and supply of, 'folk medicine' in the context of fundamental political and cultural changes in Russian society; this includes tensions and contradictions in the discourse of 'folk medicine' and the professionalisation of alternative medical practitioners.

We introduce an anthropological approach to the study of professions that highlights the significance of culture and context. We explore the dynamics here to answer three main questions:

- What is the global context for the integration of professional cultures in healthcare?
- What are the main cultural, economical and political conditions that shape the dynamics of relations between CAM and orthodox medicine in Russia?
- What is the nature of contemporary collaboration between CAM practitioners and orthodox doctors?

We draw on material from the research project on 'The dynamics of social and professional status of traditional medicine specialists in Russia', which builds on a larger project funded by INTAS, the European Union Fund for Eastern European research (for details, see Yurchenko and Saks, 2006). The research is based on a content analysis of popular medical periodicals over the last 15 years and qualitative interviews with CAM providers who practise different forms of 'ethno–treatment' (traditional forms of healing of specific ethnic origin). Here we focus on in-depth interviews with medically qualified (14) and lay practitioners (7) of CAM in the provincial city of Saratov in 2005 and 2006.

The chapter starts by discussing the global dimensions of the integration of CAM with orthodox healthcare, arguing for cross-cultural sensitivity. This is followed by an analysis of the integration of CAM services in the context of the changing Russian society and healthcare system.The findings from our interviews highlight the flexibility of boundaries between doctors and healers and the diverse strategies of professionalisation in the context of Russian culture and market-driven transformations. Finally, some conclusions are drawn on culture as a resource for professionalisation.

Integration of diverse professional cultures: global dimensions and local conditions

Scholarly debate highlights the pressures for more integrated healthcare systems in different national contexts. Changes are driven by CAM users and specialists, by business and sometimes also by official medicine. Integration may appear in the shape of unification, incorporation or subordination of CAM practices to biomedically dominated health systems (Saks, 2006). Integration may be furthered by occupational groups at the margins of biomedically centred healthcare systems that promote more flexible models of professionalisation and the permeability of professional boundaries (see, for instance, Hirschkorn and Bourgeault, 2005; Kelner et al, 2006; Kuhlmann, 2006; Saks, this volume). However, it is not only the non-medically qualified groups, but also doctors and other health professionals who may accelerate the ingress of CAM into healthcare systems, following market interests and pragmatic approaches (Shuval, 1999; Saks, 2003). Existing research highlights highly diverse strategies and interests relating to the provision of CAM services and the professionalisation of these groups. For instance, CAM specialists may use the potential of evidence-based practice and research in order to support arguments for the effectiveness and efficacy of these services (Giordano et al, 2003; Lee-Treweek and Oerton, 2003), but they may also oppose an evidence-based approach to specific therapies as it challenges a more holistic approach.

The 'incorporationist scenario' (Saks, 2006) seems to be an outcome of different stakeholder arrangements and power relations in healthcare. One key dimension that may lead to the success or failure of professionalisation is the state–profession relationship and the regulatory structure of healthcare systems (Kelner et al, 2004). In drawing on historical analysis and a comparison of Britain and the US, Saks (2003, p 89) was able to demonstrate the significance of the 'differential legal terms on which the exclusionary social closure of medicine was based'. His research revealed a more rapid move towards the integration of alternative medicine in the US as compared to Britain (Saks, 2003). Accordingly, tighter regulation together with market-driven interests may further the integration of CAM practices.

Another important driver towards inclusion is consumer demand, although it does not necessarily translate into a 'public' interest. Kelner and colleagues

(2004) assessed the views of Canadian government spokespersons on the efforts of CAM groups to take their place in the formal healthcare system. Their findings highlight tensions between the mandate of the state to protect the public and its obligation to respond to consumer demand (see also Saks, 2003). While expressing some sympathy with CAM, the interviews with governmental representatives nevertheless indicated hesitation and caution (Kelner et al, 2004). Another example is in the US where many CAM services are not covered by health insurance, although they meet the needs and demands of patients (Vallerand et al, 2003). In these circumstances, integration is especially supported by the wealthier consumers (Barrett, 2003).

A third dimension that shapes patterns of integration, and the very concept of CAM itself, is 'culture'. In Turkey, for instance, the CAM integration project conflicts with earlier modernisation policies that oppose longstanding forms of religious and political culture represented by traditional healers. This has led to its marginalisation (Dole, 2004). In drawing on Asian medicine and acupuncture, Kim (2006) directs our attention towards the interaction between traditional medicine and science and introduces the notion of 'transculturalism' to grasp hybrid formations.

Globalisation shapes the provision, content and organisation of healthcare services. In particular, the introduction of internal markets and the politics of evidence-based medicine and medical performance further the legitimation of certain types of services and the establishment of global standards and rules of conduct for practitioners. For example, Tibetan medicine is widespread in Europe and North America. Although Tibetan medicine is produced globally, it is consumed within a 'local' tradition (Janes, 2002). This illustration highlights that globalisation cuts deeply into local contexts via various flows of people, images, technologies and ideas; it enhances redefinitions of identity, suffering and corporeal practices among consumers and providers in different parts of the world. Mass consumption of local healing practices is structured by the laws of the global market, and at the same time these practices may be locally produced and consumed.

We argue that there is a need for cross-cultural sensitivity in the study of medical practice, especially the use of knowledge about illness and treatment experiences shared by a patient and a practitioner (Seymour-Smith, 1986). We can explore the cognitive and symbolic assessments of situations, symptoms and feelings that are linked to treatment practices. We have to acknowledge, however, that medicine of any type is also an ideological practice and the symbols of healing are the symbols of power.

The healthcare system in Russia: from monopoly to inclusion?

Classification of the types of medical systems suggested by Stepan (1985) distinguishes monopolistic/exclusive, tolerant, mixed, inclusive and integrated medical systems according to their openness to different healing practices. A typical example of an exclusive or monopolist system is the Soviet healthcare system, where doctors were state servants employed by the Commissariat of Health (later the Ministry of Health Care), while all other groups of healers were banned in the USSR in 1923.

Although under socialism CAM 'did not fit into modernized socialized medicine based on biomedical principles' (Yurchenko and Saks, 2006, p 110), the interest in folk medical practices, especially herbal remedies, was noted in the history of Soviet medicine. In 1919, for instance, a laboratory was established in Leningrad to study the healing properties of plants and herbs. The All-Soviet Chemical and Pharmaceutical Research Institute began systematic research into folk medicine in 1928 and, in 1931, a special All-Soviet Research Institute of Herbs and Aromatic Herbs was established, which even operated experimental laboratories in the province.

Interest in *fitoterapiya* (herbalism) greatly increased during the Second World War, the 'Great Patriotic War', due to the shortage of drugs and medical services (Kovaleva, 1972). Herbs were collected with the help of schoolchildren and teachers and subsequently processed on an industrial scale. While lay healers continued to perform their work underground, official medicine's interest in herbal treatment continued to grow. Pharmacies sold different kinds of herbs and doctors often prescribed them due to a lack of other drugs.

The rise of CAM as a means of political and cultural change

Unorthodox remedies and services started to become more widely popular in the early 1980s. Medical schools also started offering further qualification courses in manual therapy and reflex therapy. A medical counter culture emerged in Russia that mirrored earlier developments in Western health systems (Yurchenko and Saks, 2006). The growth of CAM popularity was part of a process of liberation in Russia, and the sign of a new willingness to end the mono-ideological system of knowledge and beliefs. Soviet power was on the wane throughout the 1980s and 1990s and crucial changes took place in society, leading to the transformation of the planned economy into a market economy. The healthcare system was in crisis and science, industry, technology and social services lagged far behind Western European countries. Soviet medicine was starved of resources, especially in rural areas (Yurchenko and Saks, 2006). In urban areas, patients were dissatisfied with health services and technologies and with the nature of communication with medical doctors. Queuing was a way of life at the health centres (*polikliniki*) and psychologists and social workers lacked the necessary skills to assist people with diseases, traumas and other ailments (Vein, 1990).

In this climate of change, reports abounded in the mass media that either validated or repudiated the beneficial effects of telekinesis, clairvoyance, astrology, psychic power, magic and other similar services (Romanov and Iarskaia-Smirnova, 2007). Towards the late 1980s and early 1990s numerous healers became national heroes by allegedly treating the whole population through free and accessible television and radio performances that included hypnotism, brightening water and even 'curative silences'. Such 'miracles' and 'heroes' served public demand well as a sort of 'cargo-cult' during a transitional period when the loss or painful revision of political ideals caused feelings of uncertainty. According to Vein (1990), diverse political, cultural and social movements began to surface, views became more polarised and the interests of many people inclined to mysticism.

In 1996 the Ministry of Health Care and the Medical Industry of the Russian Federation – concerned with the high risk of the mass hypnosis of the wider public – approved a statute to regulate non-traditional healing methods (Ministry of Health Care and the Medical Industry of Russian Federation, 1996), thus putting an end to curative psychics' television séances. The 'medical counter culture', however, was socialised to some extent by the earlier efforts of Soviet healthcare authorities. Official medicine in Soviet Russia had gradually opened up to CAM practices and methods, although the acknowledgement of CAM practitioners as legitimate agents of the healthcare system was still a matter of public concern and suspicion. There were attempts to replace the various healers with medically qualified CAM specialists. Yurchenko and Saks (2006) highlight that the Ministry of Health Care and the Medical Industry was willing to protect the public from 'quacks'; it was argued that 'the supply of medically qualified doctors with knowledge of CAM therapies should be increased to the point where there would no longer be demand for lay CAM therapists' (Karpeev, cited in Yurchenko and Saks, 2006, p 112).

Culture: the symbolic and social capital of CAM practitioners

Many lay folk healers oppose medical qualification per se, as it contradicts the nature of their 'symbolic capital'. Folk healers see themselves and their healing powers as part of a long tradition. This is reflected, for instance, in traditional Russian or exotic names – like 'Baba Ania' (Granny Ania) or 'Iverona Sigismundovna' – mysterious biographical facts and claims to have inherited a 'special gift', the leitmotiv in interviews with folk healers (Iarskaia-Smirnova and Grigorieva, 2006). The concept of professionalisation, generally perceived hitherto as a means to obtain 'ranking signs', such as diplomas, theoretical knowledge, status and higher wages, is reconsidered here in the context of the contradictions of the folk–urban symbolic continuum. Notably, some of the medically qualified CAM specialists emphasised their modern and 'rational' qualifications and, at the same time, legitimised their choice of practice through the roots of their family trees and socialisation – for example, growing up in a certain, usually 'oriental', ethnic community.

An official discourse has stressed that medical diplomas are important indicators of 'real' doctors as opposed to 'quacks' (Serebriakov, 2000, p 35). However, the discourse often falls short of reality (Yurchenko and Saks, 2006). As one of our informants noted: 'There are no good or bad, right or wrong methods. There are only good or bad doctors. There are more than enough frauds that have got their diploma and are working in medicine' (acupuncture specialist).

In 1993 a legal framework for regulating CAM services was established (see Ministry of Health Care Legislation, 2003). This law

> proclaimed that only medically qualified doctors who received state registration could practise CAM therapies. Only one group of lay practitioners was exempt, namely officially termed 'folk healers' who could prove that they had a special gift for healing. (Yurchenko and Saks, 2006, p 113)

The healers, too, in order to get the right to work in the area of 'folk medicine (healing)' have to obtain an official certificate and go through the authority's licensing procedures.

The debate on 'non-traditional' medicine was at the top of the agenda during the 1990s. However, at the turn of the 21st century Russian popular-scientific medical journals reported irregular renewal of, and even falling, interest in folk medicine (Iarskaia-Smirnova and Grigorieva, 2006). It is interesting to note here that the contemporary Russian medical discourse runs counter to international developments. For instance, in 2002 the World Health Organization established the first global strategy aimed at the integration of traditional and alternative medicine (Holliday, 2003).

By the late 1990s the 'industry of sorcery' had lost its democratic-missionary nature and become selectively available to different social classes of consumers. It was possible to find not only such figures as a neighbourhood fortune-teller or healer in the free-ads newspaper, but also 'corporate magicians' – exclusive herbalists with exotic diplomas working in parlours known to only a small circle of the initiated. The fashion among the political and celebrity elite thereby enabled some healers to successfully turn their symbolic capital into market power.

Demand and supply: drivers towards inclusion of CAM services

While CAM providers use the media to promote their interests (see Valente, 2003, for developments in Canada), orthodox doctors make use of their power to shape the official discourse. They predict a limited demand for folk medicine and attempt to link the provision of CAM to specific ethnic and cultural groups and/or mentally ill people, effectively reducing demand. In contrast to this, however, the INTAS project data reveal that up to half of the medical doctors working in state or municipal health services also practise CAM. Their motives for doing so are diverse, but include 'easing the workload for problems that orthodox medicine cannot solve' (Yurchenko and Saks, 2006, pp 122-3). Financial motives also play a part, as CAM services are in demand among more affluent clients, but are not included on the list of Obligatory Medical Insurance Law. Patients have to pay for these services themselves and, in addition, providers do not need expensive equipment and can even see patients at home.

However, doctors practising CAM are not only following their own particular interests, they are also responding to public demand. They are in an emerging labour market for medical professionals and take part in the new marketing strategies of pharmaceutical companies. Within the group of CAM practitioners, manual therapists, herbal therapists, homoeopaths and healers are most actively engaged in private practice. According to our interviewees, private practice can take the form of office-based specialists, specialists at a private hospital or a state medical institution, or by offering home visits with or without a licence.

Survey data from 1,500 respondents in 44 Russian regions confirm the demand for CAM services: in 2002 every fourth Russian citizen consulted CAM specialists, although only 9% said they trusted them more than those practising orthodox medicine (Fund of Public Opinion, 2002). However, the wording of the question in this survey may have heavily shaped the responses: 'Have you or have you not appealed to the services of non-traditional medicine (folk healers, herbalists [*travnikov*], psychics, etc)?'. The illustrations given of the category 'non-traditional medicine' represent the most contested areas and less 'scientific' and 'rational' forms of 'non-traditional medicine'. Moreover, the word '*travnik*' was used to define a herbalist instead of '*fitoterapevt*'. Consequently, the list of practitioners is exclusively associated with backwardness and irrationality and may well have skewed the answers. Interestingly, this report is published on the Fund of Public Opinion website under the rubric of 'mysticism'.

A broader range of 'non-traditional medicine' and less stereotyped categories was used in another survey of 1,004 respondents in St Petersburg (Goryunov and Khlopushin, 2005). This survey revealed an overall higher demand for CAM services, which were defined as 'manual therapy, herbal treatment, acupuncture, bioenergetics and natural healing methods'. Seventy-three per cent said they had consulted a CAM specialist at least once, with manual therapy and herbal therapy the most frequent. These services were seven to ten times more popular than acupuncture, bioenergetics and spiritual healing. The preferences may be the result of the cultural identity of the consumers and also mirror the supply of CAM services. According to the INTAS data on 604 medical practitioners from three different regions of Russia, the most popular forms of CAM among the medically qualified were herbalism (51%), homoeopathy (28%) and acupuncture (13%), while the least popular method was healing that was practised by only 3% of medical practitioners (Yurchenko and Saks, 2006).

Users of folk medicine have different motives, depending on their level of income. More wealthy consumers emphasise the specific nature of the healer–patient relationship, while the less affluent say they choose CAM because it is cheap, but offers healing remedies. Rich people are more inclined to follow prestigious consumption practices by having their own personal healer or a 'famous sorcerer'; such practices are increasing, especially in show business and similar circles. We can conclude that the provision of CAM services is driven by both demand- and supply-led changes. The following section further explores the latter.

Pathways to integration: flexible professional strategies and the significance of culture

Qualitative interviews with medically qualified CAM specialists provide deeper insights into professional interests and power relations that influence the integration of CAM services in the provision of healthcare. The interviews take into account the different organisational forms of providing CAM services; six participants in the study worked in state and municipal health centres, one in a medical department of an industrial enterprise and 14 in private settings.

One important finding was that most of the interviewees did not like to be called 'non-traditional' doctors; they perceived this label as derogatory and saw it as representing an attempt to separate them from the mainstream of the Russian healthcare system. They criticised the division of treatments and healing approaches as a social construction and called for the integration of different perspectives:

> 'The term "alternative medicine" depends on one's point of view. If we speak about a patient, there is no "alternative" or "not alternative" medicine. In the first place doctors have to help a patient. And we have to decide whether to use bees, to beat the drum and to conjure out evil spirits or give aspirin for headache. Irrespective of what will help, it is the result that matters. "Folk medicine"? I don't know who has differentiated between these terms! ... How can we distinguish them? All the terms and classifications are context dependent.' (Manual therapist)

CAM practitioners criticised the building of barriers between disciplines, professions and approaches in order to divide power and resources. At the same time, they stressed the differences between alternative and orthodox medicine. The interviewees stated that – in contrast to orthodox medical practitioners – diagnostic procedures are more accurate and they have more time to talk to patients. Apart from this, CAM practitioners stressed their holistic vision of 'do not just treat but cure' and paying attention to the patient's body and soul. They also stressed their distinct cultural identity, but claimed that they had a general commitment to medical ethics: 'Ethics of doctor–patient relations must be upheld whatever methods one uses' (manual therapist). At the same time, economic aspects interface with this 'moral space' and can result in different qualities of service: 'A person comes here and pays money. Thus, one can treat medicine like a product and in this case it can be of high or low quality' (hirudo therapist).

Unorthodox remedies and services were not necessarily cheaper than biomedical therapies. As Russia was entering a global market in the early 1990s, commercial networks, like Herbalife, entered the market. Some medical doctors, who might have sincerely believed in the value of herbs, actively promoted such networks. However, their 'altruistic mission' could be questioned as these doctors benefited from financial rewards from these networks. Even today, medical doctors working at health centres and clinics are involved in the advertising and dissemination of specific CAM products. Some are even part-time employees of the companies whose products they recommend and prescribe to their patients.

CAM specialists refer to culture and ethnicity in order to gain the trust of consumers and assure a high quality of service; one example is the ethnic Korean specialists who represent an Oriental school of reflex therapy. The findings of the qualitative interviews highlight how market conditions and cultural identity are merged into a specific strategy to promote professional interests.

CAM and orthodox doctors: signs of integration and collaboration

Relationships between CAM and orthodox doctors vary from acknowledgement and respect to conflict and scepticism, with a prevalence of the latter attitude. The widespread personal and professional prejudice of orthodox doctors towards CAM hampers potential successful integration. Negative attitudes are supported by fears of 'being accused of placing extra financial burdens on the patient' and a doctor 'sometimes finds it easier to send a patient to a public service' (manual therapist). Despite the overall suspicion on the side of orthodox medicine, some of our interviewees noted that doctors of various specialties refer their patients to them. However, as one therapist said, many 'people come from polyclinics with a clear diagnosis but without any referral, just on their own' (herbalist).

The attitudes of orthodox doctors towards CAM differ from one setting to another and depend on many circumstances. Important predictors for the integration of CAM are the relationships within one institution and mutual cooperation between different specialists. A herbalist explained:

> 'People come to my office from neuropathologists, gastroenterologists, allergists, paediatrics. In this polyclinic it is the official way. I write down my treatment method on their medical card.... I guess a friendly attitude is the main thing here. I think it's collaboration and trust.... Among the patients there are many doctors and their children. They are interested in the result, they continue visiting me. They show their interest, ask questions, they want to read something on the topic because it's new to them.' (Herbalist)

Some signs are emerging that point towards an increasing integration of CAM services; for instance, telephone calls from polyclinics 'that have no specialists in acupuncture, and they just ask if it's possible to refer [a patient]' (reflex therapist). Medical students and doctors doing courses in centres of non-traditional medicine and later referring their patients to that centre are another example of a change:

'Certainly, it happens but usually these are the doctors who did a course in these centres' (healer). A further sign of a change in attitude is represented by private health centres that integrate CAM services in order to offer comprehensive medical services in one place.

Integration of CAM services and collaboration between orthodox and 'non-traditional' doctors provide a number of benefits, but 'boundary work' and conflicting professional interests persist. According to one acupuncture specialist, despite signs of change orthodox doctors continue to distrust 'frauds' or 'rivals':

> 'In my opinion we have reached a step in the development of medicine when the merger of traditional and non-traditional medicine is necessary. But I don't know how much time it will take.... Official medicine and people who are at its head do not turn to us.' (Reflex therapist)

According to one CAM practitioner, 'conflicts already lie in the past but collaboration is still in the future' (homoeopath), although herbal, hirudo and apio therapists stated that they generally had good relations with official medicine.

In times of modernisation the health system's tolerance to natural products is not only related to tradition. It is also advanced by new patterns of preventive medicine that include unorthodox remedies. It is important to emphasise here that the market economy supports these kinds of CAM services in the Russian health system; wealthy consumers often use these services for the prestigious consumption of wellness, fitness and beauty services. Another driving force, however, is the limitations of orthodox medicine, especially in the field of chronic illnesses. Different market conditions and professional interests thus shape the various pathways towards integration.

Contextualising integration: diversity of professional interests and market conditions

Within the group of CAM providers, healers seem to be the most isolated group. One major area of conflict is the lack of evidence for their activities: 'One does not know what it is ... there is some concern, gossip abounds, rumours about this, arguments for and against ...' (healer). Overall, the healers were not satisfied with the level of collaboration with official doctors; they noted the lack of contact, mistrust, and ignorance of their practice and methods – even in the face of evidence of success. Collaboration depended on context and personal contacts and was usually limited to one institution.

In contrast, manual therapists were more optimistic about the future and stressed the importance of professionalisation and increasing integration. The number of professionals in this area is on the increase; and manual therapy gained legal recognition and was officially included in the list of medical specialties in 1998:

'The hardest things are in the past, I mean when a great number of non-specialists harmed many people, when manual therapy was not included in the list of medical specialties and everybody did what they wanted. Now we face a rapid development, collaboration with various related areas of medicine, … fundamental research techniques, colleagues that share their experience without concern and prejudice.' (Manual therapist)

Homoeopathy shows yet another configuration of drivers, and barriers, to integration. Most importantly, homoeopathy clashes with the interests of global pharmaceutical corporations and the provision of very cheap treatment options goes against the business interests of these companies.

The strategies and opportunities are highly diverse but in general CAM practitioners are keen to believe they can compete with official doctors. This confidence was initially nurtured by an awareness of the deficits of orthodox medicine: treatment at state institutions is seldom of high quality and the situation is aggravated by red tape and sometimes rudeness. Participants in our study were also well aware that CAM methods are acknowledged and widely applied in the Western world. They believe that developments in Russia will follow these pathways and a growing interest in CAM services will emerge by 'enlightening' people via the mass media and medical education.

Culture, integration and professional power relations

This chapter has explored the integration of 'folk medicine' into the Russian healthcare system in the context of the political, economic and social transformation of Russian society. We have introduced an anthropological approach and emphasised the notion of culture. The findings reveal that integration is a continuing process driven by various players and interests, as well as by global and local conditions. However, culture provides a 'reference point' for both the users and the providers of services. Within the configuration of demand- and supply-led changes – and professional, governmental and public interests – culture gives CAM services legitimation and may thus serve to facilitate integration in the healthcare system. Our findings indicate that collaboration between orthodox and alternative medicine and the different groups of providers is largely on the increase. At the same time, 'boundary work' needs to be undertaken and attempts to monopolise power and resources have not yet been overcome.

One novel aspect, however, is that boundaries are becoming more fluid, the strategies of professionalisation more flexible and resources for constructing professional identity more diverse. Identity is not only based on an orthodox academic community, but also on experiences in a number of different professional and institutional settings. Furthermore, the success and failure of professional services and their legitimacy depend on various conditions, in particular: successful advertising, market conditions and demand from, and satisfaction of, the target group. The majority of CAM services in Russia are commercial and can be offered in self-sustained departments of state medical institutions or in the private sector. In this situation, different strategies for advancing new professional projects are combined that are often perceived as contradictory to successful professionalisation. Our findings highlight classic elements of professionalism (state regulation, academic community and professional identity), market logic (advertising, market conditions and user satisfaction), and culture used as 'social capital'. In this respect, the research provides another example of differing pathways towards professionalisation. Developments in Russia partially mirror the strategies of CAM providers observed in Western health systems (Saks, 2003; Kelner et al, 2006) and, more generally, of new professional groups operating at the margins of healthcare systems (see also Formadi, this volume).

Culture furnishes healthcare providers with 'social capital' that may even be transformed into market power (economic capital). However, CAM providers are part of a social, political and economic power system that promotes biomedical approaches. Representatives of orthodox doctors and administrators of healthcare organisations express their 'neutrality' and tolerance towards collaboration between traditional and non-traditional specialists; health centres employ medically qualified and certified CAM specialists, and say there is no sound reason to ban holistic approaches. However, acknowledgement of CAM and its integration has still to be fully achieved, and CAM providers are marginalised in some areas. Most effective collaboration is developed within organisational settings – usually private health centres – that offer a combination of orthodox medicine and CAM services at every stage of treatment and rehabilitation.

In conclusion, professional groups use resources like culture and develop new strategies to professionalise; a 'public interest' in these services and improved collaboration with orthodox healthcare providers facilitate inclusion in the healthcare system. However, CAM specialists continue to be 'unequal partners' in a health system governed by biomedicine. Orthodox doctors may refer to CAM specialists as 'colleagues' but non-traditional medicine is characterised as 'grandma's methods'. This reflects the subordination of CAM services and their control by orthodox doctors and healthcare authorities. Consequently, culture may turn out to be a highly ambiguous resource for the inclusion of CAM services and even a facilitator of the 'incorporationist scenario' for biomedicine (Saks, 2006).

Note

[1] The project on which this chapter is based is funded by the Russian Foundation for Humanities and supervised by Professor Valery Mansurov from the Russian Academy of Sciences, Moscow. The material was gathered from 2005 to 2006 in Moscow, Saratov, Balashov and Syktyvkar. The interviews in Saratov were conducted by the authors and other sociologists at the Centre of Social Policy and Gender Studies. Particular thanks go to Olga Grigorieva, Natalia Lovtsova, Galina Teper and Tatiana Samarskaya for their valuable help with data collection.

References

Barrett, B. (2003) 'Alternative, complementary, and conventional medicine: is integration upon us?', *Journal of Alternative and Complementary Medicine*, vol 9, no 3, pp 417-27.

Dole, C. (2004) 'In the shadows of medicine and modernity: medical integration and secular histories of religious healing in Turkey', *Culture, Medicine and Psychiatry*, vol 28, no 3, pp 255-80.

Fund of Public Opinion (2002), 25 July, http://bd.fom.ru/report/cat/religion/mistika/d022909

Giordano, J., Garcia, M.K., Boatwright, D. and Klein, K. (2003) 'Complementary and alternative medicine in mainstream public health: a role for research in fostering integration', *Journal of Alternative and Complementary Medicine*, vol 9, no 3, pp 441-5.

Goryunov, A.V. and Khlopushin, R.G. (2005) 'Market of traditional medicine of St Petersburg', *Journal of Sociology and Social Anthropology*, vol 8, no 1, pp 179-85 (in Russian).

Hirschkorn, K. and Bourgeault, I.L. (2005) 'Conceptualizing mainstream health care providers' behaviours in relation to complementary and alternative medicine', *Social Science and Medicine*, vol 61, pp 157-70.

Holliday, I. (2003) 'Traditional medicines in modern societies: an exploration of integrationist options through East Asian experience', *Journal of Medicine and Philosophy*, vol 28, no 3, pp 373-89.

Iarskaia-Smirnova, E. and Grigorieva, O. (2006) 'We are a part of nature: social identification of folk healers', *Journal of Sociology and Social Anthropology*, vol 9, no 1, pp 151-70 (in Russian).

Janes, C.R. (2002) 'Buddhism, science, and market: the globalisation of Tibetan medicine', *Anthropology and Medicine*, vol 9, no 3, pp 267-89.

Kelner, M., Wellman, B., Boon, H. and Welsh, S. (2004) 'The role of the state in the social inclusion of complementary and alternative medical occupations', *Complementary Therapies in Medicine*, vol 12, no 1, pp 79-89.

Kelner, M., Wellman, B., Welsh, S. and Boon, H. (2006) 'How far can complementary and alternative medicine go? The case of chiropractic and homeopathy', *Social Science and Medicine*, vol 63, pp 2617-27.

Kim, J. (2006) 'Beyond paradigm: making transcultural connections in a scientific translation of acupuncture', *Social Science and Medicine*, vol 62, pp 2960-72.

Kovaleva, N.G. (1972) *Treatment by herbs: Essays on phytotherapy*, Moscow: Meditsina, www.kastaneda.nm.ru/kovaleva/g6.htm (in Russian).

Kuhlmann, E. (2006) 'Towards "citizen professionals": new patterns of professionalism in health care', *Knowledge, Work and Society*, vol 4, no 1, pp 59-81.

Lee-Treweek, G. and Oerton, S. (2003) 'The growth of complementary and alternative medicine: challenges for the future', in C. Davies (ed) *The future health workforce*, London: Sage Publications, pp 161-80.

Ministry of Health Care and Medical Industry of Russian Federation (1996) *On regulation of methods of psychological and psychotherapeutic treatment*, Decree No 245 of 13 June 1996, www.mednet.com/medeks/nd/245psy.htm

Ministry of Health Care Legislation (2003) *Basics of legislation of Russian Federation about citizens' health protection of July 22nd 1993*, http://nalog.consultant.ru/doc52172.html

Romanov, P. and Iarskaia-Smirnova, E. (2007) 'Social as an irrational? Diagnoses of the year of 1990', *New Literary Review*, vol 83, pp 205-26 (in Russian).

Saks, M. (2003) *Orthodox and alternative medicine: Politics, professionalization and health care*, London: Sage Publications.

Saks, M. (2006) 'The alternatives to medicine', in D. Kelleher, J. Gabe and G. Williams (eds) *Challenging medicine* (2nd edition), London: Routledge, pp 85-103.

Serebriakov, S. (2000) 'Doctors and quacks', *Health,* no 7/2000, p 35 (in Russian).

Seymour-Smith, C. (1986) 'Medical anthropology', in C. Seymour-Smith (ed) *Macmillan dictionary of anthropology*, London: Macmillan, p 188.

Shuval, J.T. (1999) 'The bear's hug: patterns of pragmatic collaboration and coexistence of complementary medicine and bio-medicine in Israel', in I. Hellberg, M. Saks and C. Benoit (eds) *Professional identities in transition. Cross-cultural dimensions*, Södertälje: Almqvist & Wiksell International, pp 311-25.

Stepan, J. (1985) 'Traditional and alternative systems of medicine: a comparative review of legislation', *International Digest of Health Legislation*, vol 36, no 2, pp 281-341.

Valente, T. (2003) 'Social networks and mass media: the "diffusion" of CAM', in M. Kelner, B. Wellman, B. Pescosolido and M. Saks (eds) *Complementary and alternative medicine: Challenge and change*, London: Routledge, pp 131-42.

Vallerand, A.H., Fouladbakhsh, J.M. and Templin, T. (2003) 'The use of complementary/alternative medical therapies for the self-treatment of pain among residents of urban, suburban, and rural communities', *American Journal of Public Health*, vol 93, no 6, pp 923-6.

Vein, A. (1990) 'About two forms of curing', *Science and Life*, no 2, p 61 (in Russian).

Yurchenko, O. and Saks, M. (2006) 'The social integration of complementary and alternative medicine in official health care in Russia', *Knowledge, Work and Society*, vol 4, no 1, pp 107-27.

TEN

Policy dynamics: marginal groups in the healthcare division of labour in the UK[1]

Mike Saks

Introduction

This chapter analyses from a regulatory viewpoint the policy dynamics of health support work and complementary and alternative medicine (CAM) in the UK, as examples of marginal groups in the healthcare division of labour. Typically, in the past, social scientific studies of professionalisation have focused on fully fledged professions, at the expense of occupational groups with a less developed professional structure – not least in the area of health. Theoretically, this applies to traditional trait and functionalist approaches more positively oriented towards professions as much as to the more critical recent neo-Weberian orthodoxy based on the interests of such privileged occupations centred on exclusionary social closure in a competitive marketplace (Saks, 2003a). This emphasis is understandable given the longstanding, well-defined and high-profile forms of corporate governance associated with the leading health professions.

In healthcare, the medical profession has been the main focus among social scientists in the Anglo-American context. It was the first health profession historically to establish itself as 'self-regulated' in the UK through the 1858 Medical Registration Act (Stacey, 1992). As in the US where similar trends occurred by the early 20th century, this allowed medicine to dominate the rest of the healthcare workforce as the subordinated occupations allied to health began to professionalise (Saks, 2003b). Although the focus is progressively changing – with growing numbers of studies of professional groups like nurses and midwives in the healthcare division of labour (see, for instance, Davies and Beach, 2000) – medicine still steals the limelight in the published literature. In the UK, this is reflected in growing social scientific interest in the policing of medicine, which has long taken precedence over the regulation of other areas of healthcare (see, for instance, Klein, 1973; Rosenthal, 1987) – especially following the recent case of Dr Harold Shipman, the serial-killing general practitioner (Allsop, 2002).

In light of media publicity given to this and other incidents highlighting poor performance by doctors, medical regulation can once more be seen to be driving change to enhance public protection – a central plank of government policy in the health arena. However, government policy interest is now spreading to other health professions, as illustrated by the establishment of the Council for the Regulation of Health Professions – now retitled the Council for Healthcare Regulatory Excellence – to promote best practice in the regulation of healthcare professionals in the public interest (Larkin, 2002). Further down the pecking order, occupations that undertake a range of health support work, but are not systematically regulated, and the related, not yet fully professionalised, body of CAM practitioners have been of rising concern to policy makers. This interest stems in part from the potential risk they pose to vulnerable members of the public. Government policy has also been shaped by the economic gains from a more flexible workforce in the public and private sector that breaks down existing patterns of social exclusion, as well as the self-interests of health professions – despite the recent government attack on them.

This chapter documents the recent challenges posed and regulatory changes made in the marginal fields of health support work and CAM, which are currently less well governed than more fully fledged health professions in the UK. In so doing, the background to each of these areas, as well as recent policies impacting upon them, are considered in more detail alongside the mainstream political, social and economic drivers of reform. This enables a number of comparisons to be drawn. In both cases the associated workforce dynamics have impacted on the healthcare division of labour, with differential moves towards professionalisation, which bring potential regulatory benefits as well as costs for the health workers concerned and the wider public.

The case of health support work

Background

Until recently health support workers have been neglected by social scientists in the UK, with very few exceptions (see, for example, Thornley, 1997, 1998). They have previously rarely figured even in the policy literature, as illustrated by the government publication *A health service of all the talents: Developing the NHS workforce* (DH, 2000a), which focused primarily on the health professional labour force. However, the author recently chaired the Steering Group for a project commissioned by the UK Departments of Health to undertake a major review of health support workers (Saks et al, 2000) – following the report by J.M. Consulting (1998) on the 1997 Nurses, Midwives and Health Visitors Act, which called on government to study in greater depth support workers employed in healthcare settings given the threat to public protection posed by the relative lack of existing regulation. The project examined the roles, functions and responsibilities of support workers employed in healthcare settings and made recommendations to the four UK Departments of Health on the extent of regulation appropriate in the interests of public protection, and the practical means of providing it, with reference to the parallel reform of social care (Saks et al, 2000).

The project involved a literature review; a survey of chief executives of NHS Trusts, health authorities, social services departments and other related organisations; local focus groups; open regional workshops for stakeholders; in-depth interviews with key players; and a website for comment by interested parties. It highlighted that there were many different categories of support workers – with more than 300 different job titles identified in the survey of employers, most of which were inconsistently employed. These included unqualified workers within mixed clinical and therapeutic teams; autonomous but unregulated practitioners within emerging professions; workers giving frontline support to patients/users in the community and their own homes; workers providing support to service users in group care settings; and support workers directly employed by service users. The definition of a health support worker in the study, restricted to the paid workforce, was: 'A worker who provides face-to-face care or support of a personal or confidential nature to service users in clinical or therapeutic settings, community facilities or domiciliary settings, but who does not hold qualifications accredited by a professional association and is not formally regulated by a statutory body' (Saks et al, 2000, p 21).

The project, which involved studying a wide span of health support workers from physiotherapy and occupational therapy aides to community healthcare assistants and auxiliary nurses (see Wrede, this volume), also revealed the difficulties of distinguishing health and social care support workers. This was because of frequent occupational crossovers given the opportunities for such largely untrained workers to move between settings, and even to hold posts simultaneously in different settings – which in some cases led to the development of cross-sector generic roles. Despite this complication, it was estimated that the numbers of support workers employed in health and social care in the UK have now grown to well in excess of one million, even leaving aside those working in the voluntary sector, about which little data currently exist (Saks et al, 2000). This testifies to their significance as these figures greatly exceed the numbers of doctors and nurses in the UK (Saks, 2003a). Nonetheless, they remain a minority group, not least because they form a predominantly female, low-paid workforce, often employed part time (Thornley, 2003).

While some such workers are becoming more professionalised – as, for instance, operating department practitioners now registered as a profession under the Health Professions Council (Saks and Allsop, 2007) – the review found that there was a relative lack of formal public safeguards for most health support workers in the UK (Saks et al, 2000). Admittedly, there are some checks against risk based on employers, professional groups and the workers themselves – such as pre-service screening and access to information about unsuitable individuals, regular structured supervision and line management by qualified staff, and continuing development opportunities. Legal safeguards linked to recruitment, employment, the termination of employment and safety at work also exist. There are voluntary registers for some occupational groups too, complementing wider voluntary registration schemes. In addition, public protection is given through various types of education and training, such as diploma and degree courses. However, in practice such safeguards are not that strong in protecting the public against risk.

This was apparent from the questionnaire responses from chief executives in the project who felt that there were significant risks to the public when health support workers were employed – with a quarter of respondents believing these to be considerable. The following three issues were highlighted in the focus groups: identifying unsuitable or dangerous people and excluding them from the workforce; problems of role definition, which could lead unqualified staff to perform tasks beyond their competence; and standards of training. The questionnaire survey suggested that, while most organisations were taking steps to minimise risks to the public, available safeguards were by no means always employed. Overall, there was a high level of agreement about the need for further regulation of health support workers, which the vast majority of chief executives who responded supported. More than three quarters of these were in favour of such measures as raising formal education levels and more pre-service checks – with strong support for a mandatory register, which was also echoed in the regional workshops (Saks et al, 2000).

Recent trends in regulation

In this light, the review recommended that a register be introduced for health support workers in the UK – in addition to standardising their occupational titles in relation to skills/competencies, improving the directions and guidance given to employers, enhancing the active management/supervision of support workers, placing a greater responsibility on employers/agencies, further informing service users about their position and rights, and increasing the training and qualifications of health support workers (Saks et al, 2000). Although it was felt that a limited register based on pre-service checks and monitoring of records growing into a more comprehensive one-stop arrangement with associated codes of ethics should be introduced, this aspect of the review was controversial. The project itself highlighted issues over the introduction of a register, including the potential bureaucracy involved, the implications for future recruitment, and its managerial location. Indeed, the high potential costs of the register to government – particularly given the low pay of the workers and limited means of smaller independent employers – may have led to the report being embargoed, despite being widely circulated in government circles.

Fortunately, the modernising government policy framework improved public protection for health support workers in the National Health Service (NHS), irrespective of the implementation of the report (DH, 2000b). This promoted everything from evidence-based practice, clinical governance, value for money and flexible careers to the enhancement of skill mix, collaborative working and the role of the service user. Moreover, from a national policy perspective, developments in professional roles and regulation, educational provision and social care had the potential to advance public protection. As health professions were increasingly being challenged at this time and their regulatory processes updated, there were opportunities for improving their supervisory role – as well as for selected groups of health support workers to professionalise. The rise of government-supported educational provision linked to occupational standards also offered growing access to the climbing frame of educational opportunity and further mitigation against risk for the public. So too in the lateral, but related, field of social care did the introduction of the General Social Care Council in 2001 in place of the Central Council for Education and Training in Social Work to protect service users, carers and the public (GSCC, 2004).

Nonetheless, in part drawing on the review findings, the Department of Health (DH, 2004) issued a specific consultation document on healthcare staff in England and Wales explicitly based on the ongoing government commitment to increasing public safety and improving quality of health. This argued that regulation can no longer be limited to professional groups like doctors and nurses. The case was made for the selective statutory regulation of health support workers by 2007 through a new Health Occupations Committee of the Health Professions Council, while avoiding unnecessary bureaucracy and cost. In parallel in 2002 the General Social Care Council published its Code of Practice for social care workers and employers, while in 2003 a Social Care Register was established with the aim of registering all qualified social workers, followed by social work students, residential childcare workers and managers of care homes – and finally support workers in social care. Employers in social care were in turn held accountable for, among other things, the knowledge and skills development of such workers under a Code enforced by the Social Services Inspectorate and the National Care Standards Commission (GSCC, 2004).

The latter reforms will doubtless have ripple effects for health support workers given the centrality to the government agenda of joining up health and social care. In this respect, the Donaldson and Foster reviews of medicine and the wider range of healthcare occupations respectively (DH, 2006a, 2006b) have now been completed, in the wake of the Shipman Inquiry (DH, 2004). While paradoxically their recommendations do not fully hang together, there is a clear public protection message in the former, which focuses on the reform of the role, structure and function of the General Medical Council, and in the latter, which calls for greater consistency between medical and other types of healthcare in increasing standards for service users. This means enhanced support for the continuing development and regulation of staff like healthcare assistants, therapy assistants and assistant practitioners in areas where there is regular contact with patients, such as radiography and rehabilitation. The corollary is that other health support workers not directly involved in clinical care like domestic, portering and clerical staff would be managed locally by employers. The speed of reform for health support workers more generally, however, could be slowed by the recommendation of the Foster review (DH, 2006b) that a pilot study of employer regulation of support workers in Scotland, with a non-statutory register, should first be evaluated.

Drivers of reform

Feedback in the consultation on the above reviews (DH, 2006a, 2006b) indicated that there needs to be fuller consideration of the options and their ramifications. Statutory regulation for some, but not necessarily all, support staff was favoured, given that it might be burdensome and reduce recruitment. Regulation of selected staff by the Health Professions Council was also widely supported. It is quite clear from the reviews and the consultation that public protection is central to the reform of health support workers, as well as the existing health professions. Even elite health professions have been under close scrutiny from the current Labour government in the more critical climate in the UK from the mid-1960s onwards fuelled by recent medical scandals such as the removal of children's organs without consent at Alder Hey and the unacceptably high rates of heart surgery on children at Bristol Royal Infirmary (Allsop, 2002).

This critical climate variously led to the replacement of the United Kingdom Central Council and the English National Board by the more accountable and transparent Nursing and Midwifery Council, and the Council for Professions Supplementary to Medicine by the less medically dominated Health Professions Council. The General Medical Council itself also had to make changes to its accreditation and fitness to practise procedures, and enhance its lay representation (Allsop and Saks, 2002). In the case of health support workers, the need for greater public protection was accentuated because such workers provide face-to-face care and support, often unsupervised in people's own homes, and therefore pose a risk to vulnerable members of the public.

Aside from the need to develop appropriate standards of practice, conduct and training for health support workers, another reason for intensified interest in policy on the regulation of health support workers is that it is now a financial imperative for government. Since the present Labour government took office, there has been a desire to contain healthcare costs while raising the standard of services (DH, 1997). Health support workers have become ever more central to this agenda in a situation of rising demand, where the salaries of NHS staff make up two thirds of all healthcare costs (Wanless, 2001). Changing the roles and tasks of more highly paid and expensively trained health professionals like doctors and nurses for cheaper forms of labour through enhancement, substitution, delegation and innovation has therefore become increasingly attractive to government (Sibbald et al, 2004). The need for health support staff to take on professional roles has been underlined by the European Working Time Directive, which has decreased junior doctors' working hours and encouraged more flexible routes through to professional and other career pathways and greater regulation of quality through clinical governance (Saks and Allsop, 2007). This provides a prime illustration of the impact of European Union law in this area in the UK.

Another driver shaping the policy reforms surrounding health support workers is professional self-interests, based on the maintenance and/or enhancement of status, income and power. These have been manifested in a number of ways despite the currently rather inclement environment for health professions (Saks, 2003b). One example of this from feedback in the consultation on the Donaldson and Foster reviews (DH, 2006a, 2006b) is that a number of health professional bodies wanted to regulate those supporting their own profession – despite the lack of a clear consensus about who should set overall standards and take ownership of them. As such, whatever the benefits in terms of public protection, health support workers can be seen to accentuate how subordinated groups are used by professions to gain additional social standing – as pawns in the battle over professional supervision and oversight (Saks, 2003a). The makeweight in this tussle for less well-qualified groups like health support workers that have not achieved exclusionary social closure is of course unionisation. However, the very diversity of these less privileged workers may diminish their effectiveness as a lobby against the relative power of the health professions (Thornley, 2003).

The case of complementary and alternative medicine

Background

The power relations between orthodox medicine and CAM have also been a familiar theme in the literature on this subject. In this sense, the current political legitimacy of medical orthodoxy contrasts with the relative marginality of CAM in the UK, which is defined by its limited representation in a number of key areas, such as in the mainstream medical curriculum, leading medical journals and official research funding. In this light, it should not be surprising that CAM shares the distinction with health support work of only relatively recently being systematically studied in the UK by social scientists (Saks, 2003b). In addition, CAM has rarely figured in recent government policy documents on healthcare – still less on the NHS (see, for example, DH, 2000a, 2000b). As with health support work, the author has also played an engaged role in raising its profile – as Chair of the Research Council for Complementary Medicine and a member of key national committees on CAM linked to the Department of Health.

Like health support work, of which certain non-professionalised forms of CAM are a part under the definition adopted in the health support worker review, it too has a major, unpaid self-help dimension – with the role of carers paralleled by direct users of CAM and their friends and families (Saks, 2003b). CAM itself also shares the diversity of health support work, which is clearly indicated by the pioneering report of the House of Lords Select Committee on Science and Technology (2000) that divided CAM into three categories. The first comprised therapies believed to have the most credible evidence and most organised practitioners – acupuncture, chiropractic, herbal medicine, homoeopathy and osteopathy. The second category was seen to complement orthodox medicine – as, for example, aromatherapy, counselling, hypnotherapy, massage and reflexology. The third group of therapies was held to have principles opposed to orthodox medicine and a less convincing evidence base – such as the longstanding health systems of Ayurvedic Medicine and Traditional Chinese Medicine, as well as crystal therapy, iridology and radionics.

This division is contentious, not least because acupuncture is placed in the first category, while Traditional Chinese Medicine, of which it is also a part, is located in the third category. However, the report certainly highlights that CAM is as complex as health support work. This is accentuated further when attempts are made to distinguish CAM from orthodox biomedicine – which is primarily based on the employment of drugs and surgery to repair parts of the body that have broken down (Saks, 2006) – by using stereotypical labels like 'holistic medicine' and 'traditional medicine'. When specific aspects of CAM are examined in more detail it is apparent that although some types of CAM approximate to these labels – such as Traditional Chinese Medicine centred on synergistic mind–body links with a several thousand year history – many others do not. Biofeedback, in which technical instrumentation is used for self-monitoring mental states, for instance, is holistic, but is of very modern origin. The employment of osteopathy simply to treat bad backs meanwhile can be very non-holistic, even if the origin of osteopathy itself goes back more than a century (Saks, 2003b).

The practice of CAM has if anything also experienced even greater growth than health support work in general over the past two or three decades from a very low base in the early 1960s. Of the 60,000 CAM practitioners now in operation in the UK on a full- and part-time basis, it is noteworthy that – with the growing exception of such settings as general practice and pain clinics – most operate in the private as opposed to the public sector (Saks, 2006). One reason for this distinction from health support workers is that CAM therapists without orthodox health qualifications are excluded from the NHS as practitioners in their own right, while orthodox health professionals who practise CAM have often seen this as a route to gaining a living in the private sector (Cant and Sharma, 1999). This further adds to the diversity of CAM practice, in so far as there are both orthodox health professionals and non-professionals involved in the field – in addition to the osteopaths and chiropractors who won their professional standing in the 1990s, and other practitioners with very limited or non-existent training who exercise their right to practise under the common law (Saks, 2003c).

Concerns over public protection in this variegated field were part of the rationale for the report of the House of Lords Select Committee on Science and Technology (2000), which aimed to inform the public and policy makers about CAM. Even compared to health support work, greater risks are potentially involved given the more restricted role played by employers in regulation, and the higher levels of autonomy of CAM practitioners, who can still operate in many areas without qualifications. It should not be surprising, therefore, that the report made various recommendations to progress the field including, among others, that:

- the NHS should ensure access to CAM through medical referral when evidence of efficacy and robust regulation exists;

- professional regulation should be developed further for CAM on a statutory or voluntary basis as appropriate;
- training in CAM should be linked to higher education, incorporating research methods and biomedical knowledge where relevant;
- orthodox health professions should be familiarised with CAM, with guidelines on standards;
- research into CAM should be extended with the support of government;
- more information on CAM should be given to the public.

Recent trends in regulation

Historically, CAM therapists were able to practise in open competition on a level playing field in the UK before the rise of a legally differentiated medical profession and the allied health professions. With further legislation in the 20th century ensuring an effective monopoly of state practice, the medical profession gained an even stronger position of dominance and CAM practitioners were progressively marginalised to the point of extinction (Saks and Lee-Treweek, 2005). This began to change with growing public demand for CAM from the 1960s onwards, despite resistance from the medical profession. This public support manifestly helped to make government more receptive to policy reform in relation to CAM than in earlier periods when the overtures of groups like the osteopaths intent on gaining professional standing were rejected as a result of the medical–ministry alliance (Saks, 2005). One of the first fruits of this was when the Conservative government of the 1980s pronounced itself keen to promote an umbrella approach to the professional regulation of CAM. However, this was not realistic given the many divisions in CAM, despite the existence of overarching bodies like the Institute for Complementary Medicine and the Council for Complementary and Alternative Medicine (Saks, 2003b).

Nonetheless, further regulatory progress was made once the government relaxed its search for a unified approach and left each therapy free to seek its own form of recognition. This ultimately led to the 1993 Osteopathic Act that established the General Osteopathic Council, which oversees a register upholding ethical and educational standards and providing statutory protection of title. This was followed by the parallel 1994 Chiropractic Act that led to the formation of the General Chiropractic Council charged with similar functions (Saks, 2006). Both Councils were created through private members' bills – and, even though neither allow the access to practise in the NHS achieved by more orthodox health professions, they do represent a step forward in the professionalisation of CAM in the UK (for a comparative picture see Iarskaia-Smirnova and Romanov, this volume). This trend among CAM therapists is stronger than that normally found among health support workers.

In spite of this, the current position of CAM therapies in the UK remains mixed from a professional regulatory viewpoint. At one end of the spectrum, practitioners of types of CAM like crystal therapy are not greatly disposed to professionalisation, reflecting their stronger emphasis on self-help and a less well-developed knowledge base. Further along the line are aromatherapy and reflexology, which have a plethora of occupational associations and schools. However, they have yet to produce a coherent approach to professionalisation and are not helped by the typically fairly short training at present. Groups like acupuncturists, however, have moved closer to achieving statutory regulation like the osteopaths and chiropractors. They currently have a voluntary code of discipline, education and ethics, to which most practitioners are signed up. Earlier rifts between a wide range of disparate acupuncture bodies were overcome following the establishment of the British Acupuncture Council, the registering body, and the British Acupuncture Accreditation Board, which lays down minimum educational standards (Saks, 2003b).

At a wider level, many of the recommendations of the report of the House of Lords Select Committee relevant to regulation were well received (DH, 2001). Several of these have been implemented – including, for instance, the government pump-priming of research into CAM and the encouragement given to the development of CAM courses in higher education. In addition, the Department of Health was one of the commissioners of two recent reports that recommended the statutory regulation of acupuncture and herbal medicine respectively (Acupuncture Regulatory Working Group, 2003; Herbal Medicine Regulatory Working Group, 2003) – in the latter case potentially through a broader CAM Council. The Prince of Wales's Foundation for Integrated Health was also centrally involved in commissioning these reports. The Foundation has since explored further regulatory proposals for CAM – including the appropriate form and mix of statutory and voluntary regulation (see, for instance, Stone, 2005) – in association with the Department of Health, which has provided substantial funding for its work in this area.

Drivers of reform

While statutory regulation in CAM still remains the preserve of the osteopaths and the chiropractors, the more recent regulatory initiatives have been explicitly driven by the desire to increase public protection. It should not be surprising that the initiatives that have been taken by the Department of Health and other parties such as the implementation of the general modernising policy agenda of the NHS – with its range of provisions from enhancing clinical governance to strengthening the role of the service user (DH, 2000b) – have a greater impact on the regulation of health support workers than CAM therapists as the latter are much more heavily concentrated in the private sector. Having said this, the proposals put forward by the Department of Health (DH, 2004) in its consultation document on the regulation of healthcare staff through a new Health Occupations Committee of the Health Professions Council have potential application to CAM therapists as well as health support workers more generically. So too do the recommendations put forward in the Foster review referred to earlier, which, among other things, called for the General Osteopathic Council and the General Chiropractic Council to be brought more into line with other health professions in terms of their formal obligations to the public, given its principal aim of protecting service users (DH, 2006b).

As with health support work, therefore, a central driver for the government's plans for the regulatory reform of CAM is the concept of public protection. In addition, there are also financial benefits to government from the rising number of patients taking up CAM therapies. Although the demand for healthcare is by no means fixed, the growing take-up of CAM on both a self-help and practitioner delivery basis in the private sector may well have reduced the uptake of services within the NHS. The potential impact of this in relation to practitioner services is indicated by a recent survey suggesting that around 22 million visits per annum were made to CAM therapists in England alone (Thomas et al, 2001). When employed or subcontracted in the NHS itself, moreover, non-medical CAM therapists are typically a much less costly and more flexible workforce than doctors, despite their higher contact time with clients as compared with general practitioners (Saks, 2006). As such, there are financial imperatives encouraging the development of appropriately regulated CAM therapies both inside and outside the NHS – even if these are less strong than for health support work as a generality with its more significant direct impact on savings in the increasingly recast division of labour in the state sector.

Professional self-interests have also driven health policy in relation to CAM as in the case of health support workers – not least in relation to the medical profession, which has had the most to lose in terms of the challenge to its status, income and power. With one in seven members of the public and tens of thousands of practitioners using CAM outside the orthodox health professions in the UK, the strategic interests of the leaders of the medical profession have shifted from outright rejection to incorporation (Saks, 2006). The position of rejection was epitomised by the classic report of the British Medical Association (BMA, 1986) on alternative therapies, which disparaged them as unscientific superstition. However, in its next report on this area, the British Medical Association (BMA, 1993) redefined 'alternative' as 'complementary' medicine and looked to find ways of working together, albeit under medical authority – such that today 49% of general practices provide some access to CAM on the NHS (Thomas et al, 2003). This capture of CAM, often itself epistemologically reconceptualised in less challenging Western medical terms, helps to explain why there has been a more relaxed approach to professional regulation in this area by the medical profession in terms of its interests (Saks, 2003b).

Conclusion

Some of the main similarities and differences in policy dynamics surrounding health support workers and CAM practitioners as marginal groups in the healthcare division of labour in the UK have now been highlighted – including the context, recent trends in regulation and the political, social and economic forces driving the policy debate on professional regulation. If anything, they have been drawn ever closer together with the publication of the government White Paper on the regulation of medical and health professionals aimed at providing safer patient care, in the wake of the Donaldson and Foster reviews (DH, 2007). This covers everything from ensuring the independence of existing regulatory bodies and the effective revalidation of practitioners to establishing a working party to determine roles that should be statutorily regulated and developing a system of regulation proportionate to the risks and benefits involved that harmonises both regulatory practice and legislative provisions. The most important specific recommendations for health support workers span from evaluating the applicability of employer-led regulation to considering demand for the statutory regulation of assistant practitioner roles based on need, suitability and readiness. For CAM as a professionalising area, the key recommendations include statutory regulation by the Health Professions Council for certain groups linked to CAM – such as psychotherapists and counsellors – and the establishment of a working group looking at the practicalities of regulating acupuncture, herbal medicine and Traditional Chinese Medicine.

Aside from being interesting in their own right, the marginal cases of health support workers and CAM therapists in the UK clearly underline the need to look outside the mainstream health professions from a policy viewpoint. At one level, they provide a compelling arena for examining incipient moves towards professionalisation. At another, they provide useful comparative material for understanding why some occupations have succeeded in professionalising while others have not in terms of the social, political and economic drivers of change. In this process, it is important to understand that there may be many potential benefits from professionalisation – including limiting the risks to clients through such mechanisms as codes of ethics, prescribed educational frameworks and research-based expertise, as well as providing access to professional privileges by the occupational groups concerned. However, there is also a downside as the current critique of more established health professions has highlighted – as, for example, the danger of creating further bastions of self-interested professional protectionism and increasing work within constraining bureaucracies (Saks and Lee-Treweek, 2005). Nonetheless, with the new checks and balances, this may be a small price to pay in an era when – for all its public service ideology – the cost containment policy of the government may itself ironically be most hazardous to the public as it seeks to achieve an appropriate skill mix in the modernised healthcare labour force.

Note
[1] The author is grateful to the UK Departments of Health for allowing the release in 2005 of the *Review of health support workers: Report to the UK Departments of Health* (Saks et al, 2000), on which this chapter is partly centred.

References

Acupuncture Regulatory Working Group (2003) *The statutory regulation of the acupuncture profession*, London: Prince of Wales's Foundation for Integrated Health.

Allsop, J. (2002) 'Regulation and the medical profession', in J. Allsop and M. Saks (eds) *Regulating the health professions*, London: Sage Publications, pp 79-93.

Allsop, J. and Saks, M. (2002) 'Introduction: the regulation of health professions', in J. Allsop and M. Saks (eds) *Regulating the health professions*, London: Sage Publications, pp 1-16.

BMA (British Medical Association) (1986) *Report of the Board of Science and Education on alternative therapy*, London: BMA.

BMA (1993) *Complementary medicine: New approaches to good practice*, Oxford: Oxford University Press.

Cant, S. and Sharma, U. (1999) *A new medical pluralism? Alternative medicine, doctors, patients and the state*, London: UCL Press.

Davies, C. and Beach, A. (2000) *Interpreting professional self-regulation: A history of the United Kingdom Central Council for Nursing, Midwifery and Health Visiting*, London: Routledge.

DH (Department of Health) (1997) *The new NHS, modern, dependable*, London: The Stationery Office.

DH (2000a) *A health service of all the talents: Developing the NHS workforce*, London: The Stationery Office.

DH (2000b) *The NHS Plan*, London: The Stationery Office.

DH (2001) *Government response to the House of Lords Select Committee on Science and Technology's report on complementary and alternative medicine*, London: The Stationery Office.

DH (2004) *Regulation of healthcare staff in England and Wales: A consultation document*, London: The Stationery Office.

DH (2006a) *Good doctors, safer patients: Proposals to strengthen the system to assure and improve the performance of doctors and to protect the safety of patients: A report by the Chief Medical Officer*, London: The Stationery Office.

DH (2006b) *The regulation of the non-medical healthcare professions: A review by the Department of Health*, London: The Stationery Office.

DH (2007) *Trust, assurance and safety: The regulation of health professionals in the 21st century*, London: The Stationery Office.

GSCC (General Social Care Council) (2004) *Corporate Plan 2004–05 to 2006–07*, London: GSCC.

Herbal Medicine Regulatory Working Group (2003) *Recommendations on the regulation of herbal practitioners in the UK*, London: Prince of Wales's Foundation for Integrated Health.

House of Lords Select Committee on Science and Technology (2000) *Report on complementary and alternative medicine*, London: The Stationery Office.

J.M. Consulting (1998) *The regulation of nurses, midwives and health visitors: Report on a review of the Nurses, Midwives and Health Visitors Act 1997*, Bristol: J.M. Consulting.

Klein, R. (1973) *Complaints against doctors: A study in professional accountability*, London: C. Knight.

Larkin, G. (2002) 'The regulation of the professions allied to medicine', in J. Allsop and M. Saks (eds) *Regulating the health professions*, London: Sage Publications, pp 120-33.

Rosenthal, M. (1987) *Dealing with medical malpractice: The British and Swedish experience*, London: Tavistock.

Saks, M. (2003a) 'The limitations of the Anglo-American sociology of the professions: a critique of the current Neo-Weberian orthodoxy', *Knowledge, Work and Society*, vol 1, no 1, pp 11-31.

Saks, M. (2003b) *Orthodox and alternative medicine: Politics, professionalization and health care*, London: Sage Publications.

Saks, M. (2003c) 'Professionalization, politics and CAM', in M. Kelner, B. Wellman, B. Pescosolido and M. Saks (eds) *Complementary and alternative medicine: Challenge and change*, London: Routledge, pp 223-38.

Saks, M. (2005) 'Political and historical perspectives', in T. Heller, G. Lee-Treweek, J. Katz, J. Stone and S. Spurr (eds) *Perspectives on complementary and alternative medicine*, London: Routledge, pp 59-82.

Saks, M. (2006) 'The alternatives to medicine', in D. Kelleher, J. Gabe and G. Williams (eds) *Challenging medicine* (2nd edition), London: Routledge, pp 85-103.

Saks, M. and Allsop, J. (2007) 'Social policy, professional regulation and health support work in the United Kingdom', *Social Policy and Society*, vol 6, no 2, pp 165-77.

Saks, M. and Lee-Treweek, G. (2005) 'Political power and professionalisation', in G. Lee-Treweek, T. Heller, H. MacQueen, J. Stone and S. Spurr (eds) *Complementary and alternative medicine: Structures and safeguards*, London: Routledge, pp 75-100.

Saks, M., Allsop, J., Chevannes, M., Clark, M., Fagan, R., Genders, N., Johnson, M., Kent, J., Payne, C., Price, D., Szczepura, A. and Unell, J. (2000) *Review of health support workers: Report to the UK Departments of Health*, Leicester: De Montfort University.

Sibbald, B., Shen, J. and McBride, A. (2004) 'Changing the skill-mix of the health care workforce', *Journal of Health Services Research and Policy*, vol 9, no 1, suppl 1, pp 28-38.

Stacey, M. (1992) *Regulating British medicine: The General Medical Council*, Chichester: Wiley & Sons.

Stone, J. (2005) *Development of proposals for a future voluntary regulatory structure for complementary health care professions*, London: Prince of Wales's Foundation for Integrated Health.

Thomas, K.J., Coleman, P. and Nicholl, J.P. (2003) 'Trends in access to complementary or alternative medicines via primary care in England: 1995-2001', *Family Practice*, vol 20, p 5.

Thomas, K.J., Nicholl, J.P. and Coleman, P. (2001) 'Use and expenditure on complementary medicine in England: a population based survey', *Complementary Therapies in Medicine*, vol 9, pp 2-11.

Thornley, C. (1997) *The invisible workers: An investigation into the pay and employment of health care assistants in the NHS*, London: Unison.

Thornley, C. (1998) *Neglected nurses, hidden work: An investigation into the pay and employment of nursing auxiliaries/assistants in the NHS*, London: Unison.

Thornley, C. (2003) 'What future for health care assistants: high road or low road?', in C. Davies (ed) *The future health workforce*, Basingstoke: Palgrave, pp 143-60.

Wanless, D. (2001) *Securing our future health: Taking a long-term view*, Interim Report, London: HM Treasury.

Part Three
Workforce dynamics: gender, migration and mobility

ELEVEN

Free riders in a fluid system: gender traps in agency nursing in Norway

Rannveig Dahle and Gry Skogheim

Introduction

In the 1980s the Norwegian public sector was subject to substantive modernisation. As in most Western countries the principles of new public management (NPM) were introduced to overcome rigid bureaucratic and inefficient systems and improve flexibility. The new managerial regimes paved the way for different professional working patterns. Deregulation and a radical decentralisation of employment practices are part of the restructuring process. Politicians and managers, in line with researchers, perceived the health workforce to be in need of flexibility and called for more outsourcing of functions and increased use of temporary staff. As a consequence, the use of contract employees was increased. However, the assumption that NPM can solve labour problems in the public sector is highly controversial. Although NPM regimes vary across countries (Sehested, 2002; Lian, 2003), a general critique is based on the underlying political spirit of liberal individualism that focuses on 'freedom of choice' and individual values. This 'freedom' may create new constraints for individuals and also have adverse effects on the organisation of care. The use of contract employees may create, for instance, a lack of continuity and a diminution of available knowledge.

   This chapter focuses on agency nurses, who constitute a new category of contract healthcare workers. Following Bates (1998), agency nurses are defined as those who have their work life organised by a private contractor, known generally as an agency, to carry out work within any number of medical institutions within the working week. The choice of becoming an agency nurse – as, for example, a contract nurse rather than a member of nursing staff at a hospital – highlights the issues involved in the controversy. Why do they choose agency nursing? Is it through 'choice' or lack of other options? The chapter starts with an overview of theories on work flexibility and its applications and moves on to explore the gendered implications of flexible work. The Norwegian context is then set out, together with findings from a qualitative study of agency nurses in Norway. Finally, conclusions are drawn on the symbolic boundaries in the nurse workforce and how they are shaped and reshaped by the changing organisation of care.

Theories on flexibility and mobility

According to Bauman (2000), flexibility and mobility are characteristics of the modern labour market and the individual worker. Since the 1970s, the term 'flexibility' is increasingly used to define the capacity to react or adapt to changes (Grønlund, 2004). The term, although itself rather 'flexible', is often associated with positive connotations. Ideally, flexible human behaviour ought to be adaptable to changing circumstances, but not broken by them. Sennett (1998) argues that society today is searching for ways to destroy the evils of routine by creating more flexible institutions.

Paradoxes of flexibility: normative assumptions and opportunity structures

Flexibility may create new opportunities that each individual can take and make use of within certain frames, which may in turn increase or decrease, and gives a sense of freedom both in work and private life (Eriksen, 2004). However, flexibility may be more widespread in the theoretical, organisational and political rhetoric of work life than in actual social practices (Olberg, 1995; Ellingsæter and Solheim, 2002). There is a shortfall of empirical knowledge of how and when flexible staffing strategies are actually used and accepted, but it is likely to vary within industries and between institutions in the public sector (Nergaard and Nicolaisen, 2002). Research studies often do not accurately distinguish between empirical and normative models of flexibility. In particular, the shifting relationship between control and freedom – which is assumed to capture important changes in the organisation of time in the new work life – is not sufficiently clarified in relation to flexibility (Ellingsæter and Solheim, 2002).

Flexibilisation of working hours has primarily been linked to demand and supply strategies. Employers in the private sector claim that increased flexibility is a precondition to survive in an increasingly intensified capitalist market and the present set of rules regarding work contracts needs to be softened (Olberg, 1995). Furthermore, strong trades unions, wage agreements and legislation against increased flexibility cause restrictions. The literature on flexible employment also differentiates between 'numerical' and 'functional' flexibility, claiming that both are guided by the logic of a neoliberal economy (Atkinson, 1994; Grønlund, 2004; Nesheim, 2004; Crompton, 2006).

Numerical flexibility is usually associated with negative values and implies a reduction in the number of permanent employees and an expansion in the number of temporary workers. Such reorganisations are likely to have consequences for all workers, but will have different implications for different categories of workers (Sørensen, 1999). Those at the bottom of hierarchies are more vulnerable to changes than those higher up. In contrast, functional flexibility is more often associated with positive qualities such as autonomy and upgrading of qualifications (Grønlund, 2004). Advocates of the latter see flexibility as facilitating specialisation in both productive activities and institutional regulations, allowing strategic choices and the positive development of productive resources. Critics see these strategies as a new form of exploitation of the workforce as they do not offer the workers the flexibility they want (Crompton, 2006). This points to the power relations embedded in the concept of flexibility.

More flexible employment practices seem to meet with individual preferences in 21st-century societies. According to Bauman (2000), the 'identity project' of the 20th century emphasised notions of stability and homogeneity, while avoiding freezing and keeping open many options is the key to the 21st-century identity project. Similarly, Sennett (1998) argues that modern workers avoid getting truly involved in their work because stability is no longer in demand. The individual capacity to readjust in a fragmented world not only is highly valued, but has even become an expectation imposed on the individual (Bradley et al, 2000). In the 'knowledge society', workers and employers alike tend to regard professional knowledge as personal, not collectively shared social capital with normative obligations (Solheim, 2002). The consequences of these broad societal changes may be lower investment in personal and professional careers and more fragmented working trajectories, which may damage collective spirit and traditional loyalties.

Flexible contract work is embedded in a complex nest of multiple meanings and material conditions. As indicated above, some professionals may have much to gain from recent developments, since the strong focus on individual freedom runs parallel to a range of new structural work options. Highly mobile careers may challenge the boundaries across various categories of professionals and workplaces, and flexible professionals may reject vertical career paths and top positions. However, even for successful and flexible professionals there is a price to pay for more individual freedom (Morgan, 1999).

Flexibility may be acknowledged as a source of inspiration, but covers constant uncertainty regarding income, stability and continuity; this uncertainty makes the individual more vulnerable to changing labour market conjunctures. Here a paradoxical effect comes into view: there may be even less flexibility for the individual, as flexibility makes everyone constantly accessible in the boundless labour market (Eriksen, 2004). This may be true of professionals and academics, but hardly describes the situation of healthcare personnel in general and, particularly, those with little or no education at the bottom of the health workforce. The paradoxical effects of flexibility may be even stronger for part-time professionals: they are more vulnerable than full-time professionals and more likely to be delegated jobs with limited possibilities for upward mobility and career building. The specific conditions of part-time work – with the vast majority of female workers – embody a gendered notion of flexibility (see also Wrede, this volume). We will come back to this issue later in the chapter.

Flexible workers: the postmodern 'strangers'

Simmel introduced the notion of the stranger who in many respects resembles the modern, flexible worker. He argued:

> If wandering, considered as a state of detachment from every given point in space, is the conceptual opposite of attachment to any point, then the sociological form of 'the stranger' presents the synthesis, as it were of both these properties. (Simmel, 1971, p 143)

Following his argument, there is a union of closeness and remoteness in this position that is to be found in every human relationship and constitutes a specific form of interaction. The mobile person is not bound up organically through established ties of locality or occupation. This free position allows the group to be confronted with an 'objective' attitude that does not signify mere detachment and non-participation; it is a distinct structure composed of remoteness and nearness, indifference and involvement. The stranger is near and far at the same time. This position points to the ambivalence of the stranger.

An agency nurse resembles Simmel's notion of the stranger in being constantly on the move, switching flexibly from one working context to another. The concept of the stranger may therefore help to better understand the complex effects of flexibility. However, as mentioned previously, flexibility turns out to be a gendered strategy when applied to the nursing workforce.

Gendering the concept of flexibility

More than 95% of Norwegian nurses are women, and women also constitute the vast majority of agency nurses. Furthermore, nursing is culturally coded as women's work and 'femaleness' is the ruling norm. Given this backdrop, changes in the organisation of care are inevitably linked to changing gender arrangements and women's work preferences in society at large. Norwegian women's entrance on the paid labour market corresponded with the expansion of the welfare state from the early 1970s, when an entirely new workforce was needed. Since most women at that time wanted to combine paid employment with caring responsibilities, the new jobs were constructed as part-time jobs – more than 70% of women in the labour market now work part time. Employers in the public sector therefore introduced part-time work and flexible time regimes to attract women at this particular point in history, as flexibility was built into the organisational structures of welfare state work.

Feminist scholars in particular have focused on women's low pay in the labour market, markedly in the caring and service occupations in the public sector. The normative model of the 'male breadwinner' in combination with cultural, ideological and symbolic conceptions of female work as less valued work is still relevant. However, there is evidence for a changing trend in women's work preferences: in Norway, more and more women now want full-time employment, but they are unable to achieve this (Kitterød and Kjeldstad, 2004; Kjeldstad, 2006). Consequently, feminist theories on women's labour market participation need to be revised.

Hakim (1996, 2000), building on preference theory, has argued that women's major commitment still remains within the home and the family rather than in employment. Since women's restricted employment rights, formerly recognised as barriers to participation, have been removed, the 'free choice' of women is a historically new situation. Hakim concludes that women's lifestyle preferences rather than their level of education predict whether they focus on career and job or on children and family life. Her arguments are much contested. One important issue is that Hakim fails to take into account the 'naturalised' organisational structures that both shape and reshape flexible part-time work, most often on the employer's terms. Women have taken on the larger part of domestic work because of cultural conventions and long-rooted historical tradition. Cultural conceptions are dynamic, formative forces in producing gendered interactions and outcomes (Davies, 1995; Bakken, 2001; Dahle, 2005a, 2005b). A flexible 'balance' between employment and caring work is resolved via the domestication of women, coupled to varying degrees with their formal and informal exclusion from the market, which locates the problem in a structural context (Ellingsæter and Solheim, 2002; Crompton, 2006).

The fact that many women, but few men, work part time profoundly genders the issue. Grønlund (2004) reports that male part-time workers in the engineering industry had considerable influence on their working conditions, while this was not the case in women's part-time care work. Many of the women's work schemes were involuntarily part time. Kjeldstad (2006) notes that even men in the female-coded sectors are constrained by the same set of rules and norms as women, a finding that also challenges theories of individual preferences. Part-time employment in health and care work in the public sector has become a pattern that is mainly sustained by the needs of the employer and not by women's own preferences (Gullikstad and Rasmussen, 2004). From the perspective of restricted working conditions, medical agencies might be viewed as one way of resolving an old dilemma in a modernised, flexible manner. Agency work may be viewed as a means to regain autonomy and self-control, thereby enabling the construction of a work/life balance on the employee's own terms.

The Norwegian context

During the last two decades of the 20th century a series of social reforms contributed to the restructuring of the health sector. The new reforms, however, have not developed logically from shortcomings in the care system. Instead, they are rooted in neoliberalism and associated with concepts of deregulation, outsourcing and flexibility. The logic of NPM, in particular, shapes public services in new ways by applying principles imported from the private sector. This constitutes a shift from an administrative to a managerial culture and from professional hierarchies to contractual markets (Vabø, 2004). Much of the literature suggests that NPM is not, and should not be, regarded as a fixed and fully established programme; rather, it is a cluster of different elements that occur in different compositions and vary across countries. Within this new regime, professional management is sometimes considered to be an obstacle to achieving the necessary changes; professionals are accused of attending to their own interests more than those of the clients and institutions with which they work.

In the Norwegian context outsourcing and privatisation of welfare services remained low for a longer time even than in the other Scandinavian countries. This process speeded up only after the turn of the century when managerial models and the principles of a new leadership became a major interest (Christensen and Lægreid, 1997). By and large, scholars have characterised this rather slow development as decentralised and pragmatic and the process has never taken the form of an 'ideological crusade'. However, the logic of the changes is that they have a certain way of ordering the elements that have to be followed up by certain other changes – for instance, quality control first, then consumer interests – in accordance with the principle of the neoliberal economy embedded in NPM.

The introduction of new managerial reforms in Norway falls into a period characterised by relatively strong economic cutbacks. Vike and colleagues (2002) emphasise that, despite this, reproductive work has not (yet) suffered – thanks to an army of committed and self-sacrificing female care workers. These women are poorly paid, but stretch themselves far beyond the claims of their formal contract in order not to prejudice patients and clients. Recruitment to medical agencies might have come from this workforce.

In 2001, for the first time, a social reform introduced the hiring in and hiring out of healthcare personnel; subsequently, medical agencies were established all over the country. The reform was part of the endeavour to modernise the public sector. The assumption was that deregulation of the labour market would increase both flexibility and efficiency in relation to staffing problems. The Norwegian Nurses Association reacted with a debate on the impact of agency work on professionalism. It was assumed that a large proportion of its members would consider leaving public health institutions and turning to private agencies – and also that, subsequently, the expanding privatisation of nursing employment might negatively affect their professional interests and professional identities. Fighting for, and assuring, the quality of care in the public sector was a core value and also a constituent of their self-image. The fear of losing a grip on the situation, however, was not borne out. Later statistics showed that less than 1% of the 91,300 Norwegian nurses actually made the new private agencies their new workplace (Norwegian Board of Health Supervision, 2006).

One reason for this low move towards agency work may be the specific conditions of the medical agencies. In nursing, these are based on qualified specialists to ensure the quality of services, where employment is without exception based on a minimum of two years' post-education work experience.

The situation is markedly different from other agency workers in the new labour market, where the majority of workers are young, low-educated women (Torp et al, 1998) and agency work is perceived as a pathway to more permanent positions and careers in the labour market (Gezelius, 1999).

The empirical study: motives and experiences of agency nurses

Agency nurses – although only a small category of Norwegian nurses – provide an interesting case study to highlight new tendencies in the NPM-driven health sector. Empirical data from a larger project financed by the Norwegian Research Council serve to illuminate these issues. The project aimed to explore the implications of the 2001 public sector reform. Key research questions were:

- How do medical institutions use the new agencies?
- What are the implications of the reform at the ward level?
- What are the motives for and experiences of being an agency nurse?

In the following, we will focus on the third question and the associated interview material. All interviews were undertaken three years after the implementation of the law. The sample comprised 16 agency nurses, comprising 15 women and one man. One criterion for participation in the project was that the agency had served as their main employer; another was that participants should have worked both in hospitals and agencies long enough to have some significant experiences. Except for one, all of them were recruited through agencies.

Why work as an agency nurse?

At the point of implementation of the law, many of the Norwegian nurses were frustrated, exhausted and even outraged. Major complaints were tough working regimes, limited control over working conditions and low wages in relation to doctors. Turning to an agency implied a considerable wage increase compared to employment in a medical institution, as one nurse explained: 'I was well educated and really strived for better pay. What was the point? Nursing means hard work and lots of responsibilities' (B1). She acted for her own individual good, while another nurse took a collective perspective into consideration: 'Our Association has always cried out for more pay, but they will never succeed as long as they do it collectively. I think that the agencies might be helpful to create a challenge' (B2).

In the annual assembly meeting in 2001, the Nurses Association recognised that the reform had come into practice and the case was lost. Members were therefore encouraged to make strategic use of the agencies to improve wages for all. Agency nurses might thus serve as spearheads in wage negotiations. While a fighting spirit was a strong leitmotiv to some nurses, others were resigned to their lot. A high workload over a long period was often caused by a series of organisational changes:

> 'Two wards were united, but this didn't work well and very little was done to support the staff. The ward was constantly overloaded and people almost died in our hands while we were lacking the resources to handle these situations. I had good relationships with my colleagues but I was worn out and just had to quit.' (B11)

While this feeling was related to a structural problem in the workplace, other interviewees aimed at a better work and private life balance: 'I felt so stuck in a rigid shift regime and wanted shorter working periods. So I would try to work a little here and there and just see how I like that and whether I feel more free' (B2).

All these decisions were related to discouragement and a protest against a rigid work regime that encouraged a sense of being disregarded, personally as well as professionally. Some interviewees hesitated as to whether agency work really was a better working option, while several others clearly felt that it provided better opportunities for combining work and family commitments. The latter judgement was often underpinned by traditional female core values and the cultural script of being a 'good mother'. For instance, one nurse did not want to work in the evening as she felt guilty about leaving her children alone – even when the father was present.

Other motives to choose agency work were to broaden professional horizons. One young nurse explained:

> 'Agencies offer a perfect alibi to see more, and on the CV it doesn't look as if you were an unstable person. I want to try many different things, but I cannot work half a year here and half a year there, that would not make me look serious. I can only do this through agency work.' (B6)

In a position as a 'wanderer' she could pick and choose, and agency work expanded her range of opportunities for creative career planning. An experienced elderly nurse with grown-up children felt free to do whatever she wanted. Being a wanderer was a golden chance to fulfil her dream of travelling all over Norway. Frequently receiving information from her agency, she was able to look at interesting alternatives. Based on these opportunities she made up her own annual scheme of working.

Working experiences

Gezelius (1999) found that the practices of using agency workers varied between industrial companies, as did the procedures for how to receive the newcomers, when most of them lacked relevant experience. What makes agency nurses different is that they are experienced professionals with the same educational background as other staff members. Hence they are peers with a compatible competence to observe, make judgements and undertake care work, but still remain institutional strangers without knowledge about local contexts, people, routines and practices.

Agency workers are regarded as high-budget costs and medical institutions therefore seek to restrict their use to a minimum. The agencies are commonly recruited at the very last moment, when all other staffing options have failed. Consequently, there is no time to give all the relevant information needed. In one ward it was even made explicit that no initial information should be given; the agencies were expected to handle this. Part of the contract between the agency and the ward is that the agency is responsible for paying for the time needed for providing practical information, while the employer is responsible for giving the information. However, these procedures often failed and a shortage of relevant information was the most frequent complaint:

> 'You don't find the equipment, nothing is explained to you; you do
> not even get fire instructions ... I think it is indefensible the way it is
> in many places. Mostly things go well, and perhaps there are not so
> many acute situations.' (B13)

To work as an agency nurse in changing environments demands high social competence. Among other things, social competence is the capacity to be context sensitive and having the ability to adapt quickly. The lack of formal procedures, like being introduced and welcomed to a new work situation, requires high individual competencies. For instance, interviewees reported that they had to take full responsibility for introducing themselves to the ward, finding out about the routines and taking on the tasks delegated to them. However, even if not officially welcomed, the agency nurse is rarely exposed to the open, negative sanctions that are reported in studies of other agency workers (Gezelius, 1999). Most of them felt warmly welcomed, because the existing staff were relieved of a heavy work burden. At the same time, they rarely felt themselves to be fully included members of the peer group; they remained strangers in implicit and often subtle ways.

Similar routines do exist across different wards, but they are adjusted to the specific tasks and the kinds of illnesses and category of patients the ward has to deal with. To collaborate properly with the rest of the team members, the agency nurse needs to attune herself to the rhythm in the ward. She belongs to the collective, and at the same time, she is an outsider. The permanent staff set the stage as to how to work in the ward. The agency nurse works on their turf and rarely challenges the local standards and norms.

Simmel (1971), who was concerned with the boundaries between the insider and the outsider, discussed this ambivalent position. The stranger, he noted, must learn how to present himself or herself in any given context, to be sensitive to the rights and obligations of each individual, and to know what should be said and what should remain unsaid – and how to appear as an individual, but also to act as a member of the collective. The stranger is undifferentiated and constantly in an isolated position. Simmel himself did not use the term 'visibility', but there is always a risk that the stranger becomes either too visible or invisible in the team. Several interviewees highlighted this problem:

> 'Being an agency nurse, you learn how to walk carefully, you really have to. You see things that need to be worked on and changed, but you don't say anything.' (B4)

> 'I have no right to interfere in their routines, if they themselves are satisfied with them. You are not in a position to criticise; rather you should be humble and do the tasks you are delegated.' (B5)

An example of this behaviour brings the potential risks to patients and negative impact on the quality of care into view:

> 'In a nursing home there were four patients with rather big bedsores that had to be cared for. I got no report, but discovered this incidentally, since the patient complained of pains when I came with some tablets. There was a huge bedsore that had not been dealt with in three days [and this may lead to life-threatening infections]. This is the way it is.' (B8)

Having observed what she found was poor professional practice, this nurse felt unable to intervene due to her position as a stranger and lack of support from others. The statements highlight the subtle, but powerful boundaries that should not be transgressed. Agency nurses were afraid of negative sanctions if they tried to intervene in the routines of the ward: 'Some agency nurses set out to reorganise the work in a ward that was quite new to them. Well, such efforts are rarely well received and the staff may easily judge all agency nurses on that ground' (B7).

Acting without being sensitive to the subtle boundaries of the institutional fields may cause negative effects not only for the individual, but also for the collective position of agency nurses in the system of care. As a consequence, agency nurses often decide to carry out work in a discrete and adaptive manner. They are usually not integrated in the working community in the wards and have no access to professional meetings; opportunities for participating in the professional discourse are thus very limited. Being regarded as short-term workers makes them simultaneously privileged and vulnerable. The agency nurse has to be highly competent, independent and flexible to cope with the expectations of constantly changing situations. Some agency nurses explicitly aimed at constructing themselves as strangers to avoid too heavy workloads and responsibilities, which legitimated their focus on face-to-face caring work for patients. This gave them a sense of freedom and detachment, as discussed by Bauman (2000) and Sennett (1998). However, the immediate feeling of release might evaporate over time (Morgan, 1999). One statement suggests that a long-term effect might be different from the initial feeling of relief: 'It is mentally hard to make rapid shifts. Over time, you smile and learn to say, hello, it's nice here and then you say goodbye again' (B12).

Male agency nurses

The gendered implications of agency nursing have not been explored from the perspective of male nurses. Our data, and an overall very low proportion of male nurses, do not allow for an accurate comparison of male and female nurses. However, our one example points towards important differences not only in their motives and experiences, but also in the construction of boundaries. The only male agency nurse in our sample was a student who financed his university studies and experienced his position as a very good mix of two completely different worlds. When he was tired of theoretical studies, he was full of energy to do practical work. He was well received at whatever department he arrived and was genuinely interested in nursing – indeed, his positive attitude might have influenced the environments in which he worked. He often got long-term assignments. He felt accepted in the team, participated in the professional discourse and his opinions were seriously taken into account. In the interview he never hinted at any subtle boundaries of being a stranger or the feeling that he did not belong to the ward.

It is hard to say whether this perception is a result of lack of sensitivity of subtle boundaries or actually based on social inclusion. Only one experience was reported by the interviewee that supports the assumption of agency workers as strangers who should not intervene in the rules and routines of a ward: he had tried to change a few routines and introduced new ones while the nurse in charge was away – for example taking a patient out for a daily walk – and subsequently, was strongly criticised. However, our male interviewee did not take the consequences into account, while the women adapted their behaviour.

Flexible work in times of new public management: new boundaries

This chapter has aimed to move beyond the discourse of flexibility and opportunity structures of agency work in the wake of NPM regimes, in particular the 2001 social reform. The findings of our study highlight that most of those who have chosen this alternative sought better wages, more freedom and an improved work/life balance. Individual motives and working experiences of the nurses reveal a more complex picture. Agency work is embedded in a nest of multiple meanings and material conditions. This kind of flexible work may have some appeal, but becomes demanding over time. Being on the margin makes the agency nurse both an insider and an outsider to the professional peer group and draws them into a potentially vulnerable position.

The concept of the stranger of Simmel (1971) has helped to bring into view the subtle and symbolic boundaries between those who belong to the staff and those who do not. Detachment from both colleagues and patients is one of the implications. Another consequence is the emergence of new divisions of work in healthcare. A third, not well-studied, consequence is the emergence and reinforcement of new and existing gender 'traps' in the care sector. The linkage between part-time and agency work and women's needs and wishes to combine work and family commitments may create new constraints rather than facilitating negotiations on working conditions. There is a high price to pay for the flexibility and mobility of the modern worker. The research supports the assumption that a career as an agency nurse is likely to be short; expert information on current trends indicates an extremely high turnover of staff.

Six years after the implementation of the reform, agency work seems to be less attractive to native Norwegian nurses, while the need for such workers in the healthcare system is likely to increase. In this situation, Norwegian agencies will intensify their search for nurses from Eastern Europe and Asia. This new health political strategy needs further empirical investigation to explore the social effects of an eventual increase in the number of different ethnic agency workers in the Norwegian context. One negative scenario might be an ethnic and a professional split between the ward staff and the agency nurses (see Ribeiro, this volume). This is the opposite of a strategy making the agency nurses a vanguard to improve the working conditions for all nurses. A related issue is whether and how expanded use of agency nurses will affect the quality of nursing care. Good care, among other things, includes close interactions between professionals and communicative information skills in relation to patients.

Flexibilisation of the organisation of care, as suggested by NPM regimes, creates a number of new problems not only for the individual – female – worker, but also for the governance of care. The gendered dimension of care and agency work increasingly intersects with ethnic lines of division. The emergence of new boundaries in the care sector raises new demands for social inclusion and the management of diversity and may thus turn out as a future challenge to health policy.

References

Atkinson, J. (1994) *Flexibility, uncertainty and manpower management*, Sussex: University of Sussex, Institute for Employment Studies.

Bakken, R. (2001) *Modermordet: Om sykepleie, kjønn og kultur*, Oslo: Universitetsforlaget.

Bates, B. (1998) 'Contractual work: new production processes in nursing', in H. Keleher and F. McInerney (eds) *Nursing matters: Critical sociological perspectives*, Melbourne: Pearson Professional, pp 139-51.

Bauman, Z. (2000) *Liquid modernity*, Cambridge: Polity Press.

Bradley, H., Erickson, M., Stephenson, C. and Williams, S. (2000) *Myths at work*, Cambridge: Polity Press.

Christensen, T. and Lægreid, P. (1997) *Forvaltningspolitikk: Mot new public management*, Bergen: Institutt for administrasjon og organisasjonsvitenskap.

Crompton, R. (2006) *Employment and the family: The reconfiguration of work and family life in contemporary societies*, Cambridge: Cambridge University Press.

Dahle, R. (2005a) 'Doing the dirty work: gender and power in the health sector', in H.M. Dahl and T.R. Eriksen (eds) *Dilemmas of care in the Nordic welfare state*, London: Routledge, pp 101-11.

Dahle, R. (2005b) 'Men, bodies and nursing', in I. Morgan, D.B. Brandth and E. Kvande (eds) *Gender, bodies and work*, Aldershot: Ashgate, pp 127-38.

Davies, C. (1995) *Gender and the professional predicament in nursing*, Buckingham: Open University Press.

Ellingsæter, A.L. and Solheim, J. (eds) (2002) *En usynlig hånd? Kjønnsmakt i moderne arbeidsliv*, Oslo: Gyldendal Akademisk.

Eriksen, T.H. (2004) *Røtter og føtter: Identitet i en omskiftelig tid*, Oslo: Aschehoug.

Gezelius, L. (1999) *Å tjene to herrer: Vikarene mellom byrå og bedrift*, Oslo: Fafo-rapport no 318.

Grønlund, A. (2004) *Flexibilitetens gränser*, Umeå: Borea Bokförlag.

Gullikstad, B. and Rasmussen, B. (2004) *Likestilling eller omstilling? Kjønnsperspektiver på modernisering i offentlig sektor*, Trondheim: NTNU Rapport STF A04501.

Hakim, C. (1996) *Key issues in women's work: Female heterogeneity and the polarisation of women's employment*, London: Continuum.

Hakim, C. (2000) *Work–lifestyle choices in the 21st century: Preference theory*, Oxford: Oxford University Press.

Kitterød, R.H. and Kjeldstad, R. (2004) *Foreldres arbeidstid 1991-2001, belyst ved SSB arbeidskraftundersøkelser, tidsbrukundersøkelser og levekårsundersøkelser*, Oslo: Statistisk sentralbyrå, Rapporter 2004, 6.

Kjeldstad, R. (2006) 'Hvorfor deltid?', *Tidsskrift for samfunnsforskning*, vol 47, no 4, pp 513-44.

Lian, O. (2003) *Når helse blir en vare*, Kristiansand: Høyskoleforlaget.

Morgan, D. (1999) 'Arbeid og maskulinitet i endring', *Kvinneforskning*, no 3, pp 41-59.

Nergaard, K. and Nicolaisen, H. (2002) *Utleie av arbeidskraft: Omfang og utvikling*, Oslo: Fafo-notat 17.

Nesheim, T. (2004) '20 år med Atkinson-modellen: åtte teser om 'den fleksible bedrift', *Sosiologisk Tidsskrift*, vol 12, pp 3-24.

Norwegian Board of Health Supervision (2006) *Annual supervision report*, www.helsetilsynet.no

Olberg, D. (1995) *Endringer i arbeidslivets organisering*, Oslo: Fafo.

Sehested, K. (2002) 'How the new public management reforms challenge the roles of professionals', *International Journal of Public Administration*, vol 25, no 12, pp 1513-37.

Sennett, R. (1998) *The corrosion of character: The personal consequences of work in the new capitalism*, New York: W.W. Norton.

Simmel, G. (1971) *On individuality and social forms*, Chicago, IL: University of Chicago Press.

Solheim, J. (2002) 'Kjønn som analytisk nøkkel til kultur', *Tidsskrift for samfunnsforskning*, vol 43, no 1, pp 106-17.

Sørensen, B.Å. (1999) 'Arbeidslivsforskningens utfordringer til kvinneforskningen: retorikk og lokal virkelighet i det "nye" arbeidslivet', *Kvinneforskning*, no 3, pp 50-69.

Torp, H., Schøne, P. and Olsen, K.M. (1998) *Vikarer som leies ut: Hvem er de oghvilke arbeidsvilkår har de?*, Oslo: Institutt for Samfunnsforskning, Rapport 98:11.

Vabø, M. (2004) 'Effektivitet og kvlitet i omsorgstjenesten – en drakamp mellom nye og gamle styringsidealer', in R. Dahle and K. Thorsen (eds) *Velferdstjenester i endring: Når politikken blir praksis*, Bergen: Fagbokforlaget, pp 195-222.

Vike, H., Bakken, R., Brinckmann, A., Haukelien, H. and Kroken, R. (2002) *Maktens samvittighet: Om politikk, styring og dilemmaer i velferdsstaten*, Oslo: Gyldendal Akademisk.

TWELVE

From health to tourism: being mobile in the wellness sector in Hungary

Katalin Formadi

Introduction

With people's growing desire to be healthy, fit and environmentally sensitive, wellness is becoming increasingly popular as a concept. This constitutes a motivation for a certain type of tourism: health and wellness tourism (HWT). In Hungary, spas represent an important element of this sector, which has been rapidly expanding to serve a (Western) European market. Professionally organised spas are based on trans-sectoral employment and – ideally – employees have experience in both the health and tourism sectors and have tourism and management competencies. No standardised occupational profile exists in the sector, however, and there is a lack of data on employees' professional backgrounds. The as yet 'free-floating' HWT sector thus provides an exciting opportunity to investigate how cross-mobility may translate into the rise of a new professional project.

This chapter explores the patterns of movement, the strategies of employees' mobility and career pathways in the HWT sector. The analysis is based on material from an exploratory study and includes various human, organisational and social factors that either enable or hinder career development. I combine approaches from the sociology of professions and sociology of work with career studies, arguing that the professionalisation of an occupational field determines the career possibilities of employees. While the emerging HWT sector cannot provide well-defined organisational career pathways, it may offer employees more freedom in managing their careers and lives.

I start with some theoretical considerations and move on to present a theoretical and methodological approach applied to the study of the HWT sector. This is followed by empirical findings on professional competencies and career moves in this sector, especially emphasising individual demands on professional 'independence' and 'autonomy' and 'work/life balance'. The conclusion attempts to understand the meaning of being a professional in a fluid occupational field.

Professionals, 'entreployees' and careers – theoretical connections

Within the emerging HWT sector the workforce crosses the boundary between an occupation and a profession, and explores its own mobility paths and career options (see Ladkin and Riley, 1994, 1996; Ladkin et al, 2002). It may therefore be a fruitful approach to connect different theoretical approaches. According to Hughes (1958), an occupation implies a set of social relationships that provides a form of social identity. It places a person in a social context and also carries assumptions about the level of education. However, as Evetts (2003a, p 400) argues, Hughes' interest was to explore 'the differences between professions and occupations as differences of degree rather than kind'. Furthermore, the concepts of both occupation and profession have undergone change.

In classic structuralist-functionalist approaches the occupation–profession continuum served to define levels of professionalisation based on professional attributes and norms (Hall, 1994; Auster, 1996). Another theoretical strand considered a profession as a set of role relationships between experts and clients (Montagna, 1977). Since the 1970s the emphasis has been on power relations and knowledge. In drawing on the medical profession, Freidson (1986, 2001), for instance, explores the processes of gaining power and autonomy and the role of professional self-regulation. Another strand of the literature, following Abbott (1988, p 8), defines professions as 'exclusive occupational groups applying somewhat abstract knowledge to particular cases'.

More recent work puts greater emphasis on shifts in the concept of professionalism, the fluidity of boundaries, the different ways to professionalise and the varieties of professional projects (Evetts, 2003b; Saks, 2003). For example, Hanlon (1998) directs attention towards new forms of commercialised professionalism (see also Boyce, this volume). Evetts (2006, p 139) underlines that the concept of professionalism 'is increasingly used in a diverse variety of work, occupational, organisational and institutional contexts' and introduces a distinction between organisational and occupational professionalism. Organisational professionalism is characterised by managerial control of work, hierarchical structures of authority, accountability and standardised work practices and is based mainly on occupational certificates and training. Occupational professionalism involves more independence in decision making and a more collegial form of authority and is based on trust, both on the part of the client and the employer, and education, training and occupational socialisation (Evetts, 2006).

The new discourse on professionalism points to a need to link the occupational and organisational levels of work to the individual level of the actors involved. A more flexible theoretical approach may emerge that is better able to grasp the fluidity of boundaries and working patterns, as well as mobility within and between branches. Consequently, new directions in the sociology of professions provide new ways to research a 'free-floating' field, like the HWT sector with its wide range of differences in required skills and competencies, as well as in specialisms within the sector and across countries. Furthermore, recent work addresses issues of work arrangements, such as flexibility, autonomy, independence, diversity and gender relations. 'Beside the question of *what* work is done, it is significant *how* this work is done and in what specific settings' (Kuhlmann, 2004, p 79, emphasis in original). This leads us to connections with the sociology of work.

The concept of 'entreployee'

The concept of entreployee – developed in the context of the sociology of work in Germany – may also open up a new opportunity for an integrative interpretation of the terms 'occupation' and 'profession'. Addressing the structural changes in economy and society, Voß and Pongratz (1998) argue that a substantively new form of employment is emerging due to a decline of stability associated with long-term contract employment. Following their argument, there is a shift away from the Taylorist distinction between managing (profession) as opposed to implementing (occupation) work. Characteristic of the new entreployee is

> to free up the usual boundaries of the traditional employee in the workplace in nearly all dimensions – time, space, content, qualifications, cooperation etc – and enhance their own responsibility through strategies of increased flexibility and 'self-organisation' in the workplace. (Voß and Pongratz, 2001, p 241)

The first key feature of the entreployee is self-controlled work that is naturally based on a high level of independence. Employees are more committed to their jobs if they have the authority to make decisions in the work process and a higher level of autonomy in day-to-day work (controlling resources, time or in choosing projects and tasks), where 'only' the outcome is supervised. This, in turn, impacts on the level of responsibility and introduces internal competition between employees. Applying an entreployee style of management establishes market mechanisms in the organisation. The attitude towards the entreployee is described as follows: 'You will stay only as long as you prove that you're needed – by making profits' (Voß and Pongratz, 2001, p 245). The result is a higher level of 'self-commercialisation'; entreployees need to 'advertise' their competencies and make themselves 'indispensable' to the employer. A further consequence of higher levels of independence is an increasing demand on continuing professional development.

The new demands on self-commercialisation and continuing education relate to another key feature of the concept of the entreployee, namely work/life balance. The authors argue that entreployees voluntarily subordinate their private lives to the requirements of work. The entreployee needs a new form of self-rationalisation and self-determination in their daily life and work schedule; work and life cannot be strictly separated. The authors describe the new demands as follows: 'We need you totally, exclusively, anytime and anywhere, so you will have to manage your life perfectly. We want people who are completely under control!' (Voß and Pongratz, 2001, p 246). Competing in the occupational sector may call for the sacrifice of resources from the private sphere, both in material and temporal terms.

Career pathways

The new characteristics of work raise the question as to whether cross–sector occupations lay out specific career pathways. Career is defined as a 'morally neutral vehicle for describing occupational progress, or the lack thereof' (Schein, 1984, p 72). However, the concept of career not only refers to the sequence of jobs throughout the lifecourse; it is also 'a sequence of social positions filled by a person throughout their life' (Watson, 1995, p 127). The literature discusses two approaches to studying careers: the outsider/observer and the actor approach, sometimes called the 'objective' (external) and the 'subjective' (internal) career (Van Maanen and Schein, 1977). The 'objective' career approach involves a series of role transitions of the individual as viewed by an outsider (Guerrier, 1987). It can be measured by the status and prestige of the job, income and other measurable incentives and the position of the individual in the hierarchy; this is viewed as an organisational career.

Role transitions always involve crossing a series of different types of boundaries, for instance up and down movement in the organisational hierarchy or lateral change from one type of work to another (Schein, 1971). Guerrier (1987) further developed this approach with respect to geographical boundaries (national/ international relocation of jobs). The boundary concept has been criticised because it is said to lead to the misinterpretation of the nature of the career and necessarily suggests objective directions of success and failure (Gattiker and Larwood, 1988). One of the possible answers to this problem is to apply a multidimensional methodology.

The second perspective, the 'subjective' or individual career (see Collin, 1986), refers to how individuals perceive their lifecourse, how they describe their conditions of life and their actions, and how they judge their occupational progress or any other changes. This includes attitudes on professional development and perceptions of career opportunities and the advantages of a particular job. A further important dimension is individual autonomy in the development of a career strategy. The individual's career criteria are considered as non-measurable job characteristics to be placed in the context of other life spheres. Individual and organisational dimensions of a career are therefore interconnected in complex ways (Guerrier, 1987). Added to this, macro-level and structural dimensions – like the boom or decline of a sector – lay out specific pathways and shape individual career options (see also Strauss, 2001).

Researching an 'unsettled' workforce in a free-floating sector: theory and method

Following the strong surge in demand for wellness services, demands for new skills and professional services have arisen, some of which are in a process of institutionalisation. Spas play an important role within the wellness sector in Hungary, and more generally in Central Europe. For this reason, this empirical study focuses on spas. In all, 11 spas were included in the study; six of them have longer market experience and five were more recently established (since 2000). Five of the spas in our study focus exclusively on health-related services; on average a spa had 109 employees, although this number ranged widely. Participants in the study were on average 37 years old and two thirds were women; this mirrors the mainly female-dominated HWT sector in Hungary.

Interviews were carried out with two groups of employees: the employees responsible for human resource management were interviewed in depth about the health and wellness tourism job profile and the required competencies. This was complemented by 32 biographical interviews with employees working in various spas; the sample included both 'frontline' and 'background' workers and those working at the managerial and the implementation level, with a focus on career paths. A semi-structured questionnaire was used in relation to the following topics: educational background; commitment to the HWT sector; future interests and activities; and perception of career opportunities. Analysing the careers of those already employed in the field, the study explored how employees in various spas got to where they are today.

Conceptualising an 'unsettled' workforce

One of the most important differences in jobs in tourism is whether the employee has 'daily contact with guests', which we call frontline, or does their work 'in the background'. Figure 12.1 assigns participants to one of three positions: a frontline position with contact with guests (2) and background positions either in management (3) or implementation (1). Each of these groups has specific resources. One novelty of the HWT sector is a distribution of these resources that is not fully congruent with the hierarchical order between management and implementation or between background and frontline workers. For instance, contact with guests offers a series of benefits: employees gain knowledge of the guests as a form of 'human capital'; they may also receive tips and accumulate sociocultural benefits, like acknowledgement, loyal clients or even friendship. Informal benefits may motivate employees to provide a good service and 'give their best'. Interactions with guests differ from day to day and therefore the content of work is diversified. In this situation, the employee's personality significantly impacts on the nature and quality of the service and, as a consequence, shapes the satisfaction and overall experience of the guest – whether a tourist, a customer, or even a patient.

Figure 12.1: Employee groups in the health and wellness tourism sector

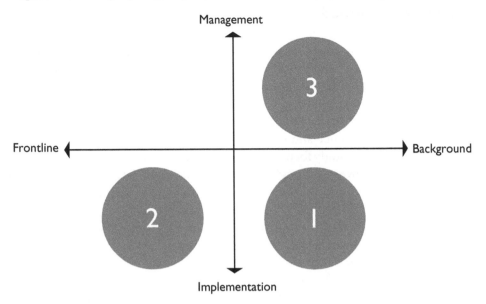

The background workers (1) are a heterogeneous group that includes cleaners, kitchen staff, technicians, administrative staff and marketing assistants. Employees in this group therefore possess very different professional skills and demands on knowledge and skills are also diverse. However, an important common feature of this group is that employees do not have the chance to develop highly valued and important skills, competencies and acquaintances stemming from day-to-day contact with guests. This is often reflected in a lack of acknowledgement or even respect for the work of these employees, especially as, to a certain degree, the person carrying out the job is interchangeable. In their work, background blue-collar workers are often faced with routine processes and monotonous tasks. Little or no interaction with guests leads to a decrease in motivation. However, this group without regular contact with guests needs further differentiation. In contrast to blue-collar jobs, the upper-level managerial professions (3) benefit from other resources of prestige and power apart from contact with guests.

Conceptualising flexible work arrangements: autonomy, control and work/life balance

When applied to tourism, the concept of entreployee needs further investigation (for a feminist critique see Henninger, 2003). The extent to which this concept and management style can be applied varies among the three main groups of employees outlined above. In the group of frontline employees, the decentralised knowledge required for the employee–guest interaction necessitates higher levels of autonomy and self-control. The management specifies aims and objectives, like quality guidelines, but employees decide how best to implement these to meet objectives. Goals and motivation, incentives and benefits within this group of employees are closely related to interactive employee–guest relationships, both financial (like tips) and non-financial (like friendships). Service provision depends on both the provider (employee) and the user (guest) and the interactions between them.

One consequence of the connectedness between provision and consumption and the significance of interactions is the replacement of central command-and-control regimes with more hybrid forms based on control by the guests and self-control. However, blue-collar employees at the bottom of the hierarchy, who have little or no autonomy, experience various forms of control, such as managerial and guest control, even though they have to take full responsibility for their performance. The situation is markedly different in the group of background employees. Whereas some of the managerial positions function along the lines of the typical entreployee described by Voß and Pongratz (2001), a great deal of autonomy and attractive incentives are combined with high levels of responsibility.

Another facet of the concept of entreployee is that employees increasingly subordinate life to work, which has inevitable effects on the individual career. Employees – mainly those interacting regularly with guests – face ongoing demands for better-quality services, new services and diverse market conditions. In this situation, successful market protection and expansion call for continuing development of skills and knowledge, and an overall priority of work commitments. These pressures do not primarily derive from the demands of employers, but rather from employees themselves who prioritise work over leisure, family and even health issues and do not wish to reduce their work efforts.

In frontline jobs the correlation of work and leisure is even stronger, as the personality of the employee is an integral part of the service provision. Tourism is often described as a 'host–guest' relationship – a business that requires the full personality of the employee to be permanently at the disposal of the guest, at any time. Although this situation is more strongly associated with traditional frontline jobs, many of the former background activities are increasingly being made 'public' – for instance, the cook working in the display kitchen. Beyond mere professionalism, 'show business' is thus becoming part of the job requirements – irrespective of the employee's emotional mood and condition. The blurring of boundaries between 'public' and 'private' spheres puts new pressures on employees and calls for new competencies of 'managing emotions' in the occupational field.

Taken together, the autonomy and flexibility of employees are connected in complex ways with occupational demands and career options on the one hand, and self-control and work/life balance on the other (see also Dahle and Skogheim, this volume). One major connection is 'time': employees may face longer working hours in peak seasons due to higher demand. Longer working hours impact on family life and leisure activities in ways that shift the work/life balance towards the demands of the job. Consequently, degrees of autonomy, self-control and flexibility are important characteristics of an employee's status in the HWT sector; further criteria of status are stability of the job contract and long-term employment, both highly valued in a branch dominated by seasonal and economic cycles.

Professionalisation and career paths at the crossroads of health and tourism: empirical findings

All employees working in the spas included in the study hold a General Certificate of Secondary Education. Interestingly, only one third of the participants in the study completed any courses in tourism, while another third attended tourism or hospitality courses at the time of the research. This supports the assumption of ongoing professionalisation in the HWT sector. Mainly those in management positions hold Bachelor or Master degrees. However, even employees in higher positions did not consider their academic degrees as relevant to their current career. All participants judged training on the job and experience in the tourism sector to be more important than degrees. They perceived personal competencies – like leadership, communication skills, loyalty, and stress management – as very important characteristics of a 'good' professional.

Frontline employees, in particular, had good foreign language skills. All of them spoke German, because 90% of the main target groups are German-speaking visitors. Frontline work proved to be an area where market relations are more important than official certificates. Most of the employees had very good conversational skills, which were used on a daily basis, without certification through an accredited language examination. Next to German, English was the second most common language followed by French and Italian, although the percentages for these two were small. Only a small number of participants had worked abroad during their studies in order to learn the language and gain international experience.

Formal certificates and special skills are only required in some areas where the field of health-related therapies is most strictly regulated. Specific certificates are required for physiotherapists, health managers and sport-recreation experts, all of whom hold higher-level jobs. All other health-related occupations such as nurses, guest entertainers, wellness therapists, fitness-wellness instructors, personal trainers, wellness trainers and wellness assistants only need a secondary education. If specific certification was required, it was usually related to the health component of the job, such as different massage techniques. Employees in more directly health-related jobs are obliged to take regular refresher courses; these occupational groups are controlled and promoted by the state.

Participants had different views on continuing education, and not all were motivated to participate in associated courses. The interviews revealed that only a minority of employees see further education as an opportunity to improve their own career development. Accordingly, professionalisation of the HWT sector is driven by new health policies and professional governance, rather than market forces and actor-based changes. Tighter regulation of the healthcare sector also impacts in the HWT sector and furthers continuing education.

Crossing functional boundaries

The findings reveal very diverse paths of entry into the HWT sector. About 20% of interviewed employees had experience in the tourism industry and worked in this sector during their studies in seasonal or weekend jobs. However, they did not think that this experience was important in bringing them into the HWT sector. Most had found their jobs through relatives or friends or job sections in newspapers. The findings indicate that most employees did not systematically plan a career in HWT, but rather entered the sector by chance. In some cases personal life conditions, like searching for a job near home, were the most important reasons for career choice. In general, neither a previous career nor the path of entry into HWT points towards any systematic effort to develop a career in this sector. This may be because of the relative lack of prestige and benefits that the sector has to offer.

Another dimension involving the crossing of boundaries was mobility and – related to this – future plans for job changes. Most surprisingly, only 25% of interviewed employees expressed an interest in changing their job, and about half of these said they would not change their workplace for a better salary or a more prestigious job. Analysis of the major sociodemographic variables reveals that the main reason for this stability is not related to characteristics of the HWT sector, but to family commitments. The majority of the immobile employees had families and children, and family relations may explain their low mobility overall, particularly when the high proportion of women in this sector is taken into account. A second reason for lack of interest in changing the job was sticking to a comfortable and accustomed life and surroundings; stability was the most important factor in the 40-and-over age group, regardless of future career plans.

Language competencies and the level of education interestingly did not predict attitudes on job mobility. Data do not support the assumption that higher levels of education and career strategies correspond with higher mobility rates. Instead, most of the employees seemed to be satisfied with the possibilities offered by their workplace and surroundings, and were not contemplating any change. Although the participants may act differently in the case of emergency – such as labour force breakdown or closure of the spa – the research does not provide evidence of subordination of the complexities of life to careerism. Consequently, the findings do not support the concept of 'entreployee' that predicts an increasing dominance of market logic and job commitments. Contrary to this thesis, the employees in the study modelled their work/life balance in favour of life.

Desirable careers

In addition to actual mobility, participants were asked to describe their wished-for careers. Results highlighted a wished-for career path from lower background to frontline and on to lower managerial positions given the opportunity in the spa where they were already employed (see Figure 12.2). This marks the general wished-for 'career track', but other pathways were also considered as desirable moves. For instance, some frontline workers would be satisfied with moving to background positions where they expected their tasks to be less controlled by guests, giving them more self-control. We must also differentiate between lower- and higher-status positions among background employees. Employees on the lower rungs of the ladder with less autonomy and independence, such as cleaners, were pleased to move to frontline positions that would offer them a more diversified job. Employees already in higher-echelon employment with higher levels of autonomy and independence, such as those in marketing and sales positions, wished to move up to management level where they expected higher positions with even more self-control and power.

Figure 12.2: Desired career paths in the health and wellness tourism sector

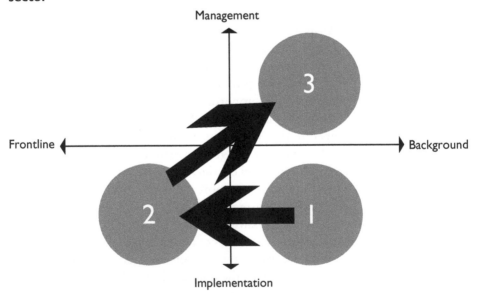

Independence in the work process

The spas in the sample were characterised by centralised hierarchy based on a two- or three-level hierarchical model: the general management on the upper level followed by employees in various departments and – usually – a hierarchical order within these departments. Employees working in financial and administrative departments had weekly meetings and had to deliver monthly written reports to the general director. Employees in marketing and sales had monthly meetings with all employees, sometimes attended by the general director. Therapy units had weekly meetings with the departmental manager, who passed on the relevant information to the general director. Physicians employed at the spas also controlled the work of employees on a daily or weekly basis. Catering units had monthly meetings with the unit manager reporting to the general manager.

Time management is an important indicator of the independence value of work. Work times were usually flexible, although certain aspects, such as opening hours, determined the working times of some employees. Within this framework, however, employees decided their own time schedule. Flexibility was highly welcomed by the management as it meant that employees could work longer than the official 40-hour week. Only a third of the employees in the study had fixed working hours. Frontline workers with contact with guests invariably faced longer working hours, including working at weekends or on days off. Despite this, these participants emphasised independence and autonomy in their job and not their longer working hours. Even in areas with more fixed working hours, employees had some flexibility. The therapy unit, where demands were more fixed by the clients, was an example of how employees managed their time schedule flexibly by changing the massage plan with colleagues and deciding on breaks.

Independence and autonomy seem to be the key dimensions in job mobility that make the occupational boundaries more permeable. From the perspective of the individual employee there are various reasons for considering autonomy to be an important feature of work. Autonomy holds out the promise of more creativity and self-control, thus offering higher psychological and social benefits. It also offers more opportunity to creatively coordinate commitments across different life spheres, and to manage work/life balance. Furthermore, the findings of the study indicate that the concept of entreployee does not encompass the complex ways in which control is exercised. Apart from a general shift from centralised command and control to new forms of self-control, there is also evidence of hybrid forms of control. Control is a dynamic concept that is applied in different ways even within a single occupational field. In the HWT sector, for instance, we found direct managerial control, mutual control between team members and control exercised by the guests.

A new professionalism in the making?

The HWT sector in Hungary is characterised by a rapidly developing market with a new workforce 'in the making'. This study looked at the cross-mobility between the health and tourism sector from the perspective of the employees, focusing on mobility, career paths and new modes of self-governance. The results provide evidence of the fluidity of boundaries between a profession and an occupation and the ongoing professionalisation of the HWT sector. However, the paths of entry are highly diverse and standardised educational programmes are not yet established. For this reason, the status and prestige of this sector are low compared to other professionalised fields and the findings of the study lead to new conclusions being drawn.

First, cross-mobility does exist between the health and tourism sector, but movement into the spas is not a systematically applied strategy. The interviews with participants in the study make clear that the sector's employees are not fully aware of the advantages stemming from the fluidity of boundaries between health and tourism. More surprisingly, although employees cross the borders of the two occupational fields, job mobility is very low overall; instead, the interviewees expressed a preference for stability. The individual strategies are also not systematically linked to career. Employees are interested in additional training courses and professional development, but the main motivation is to fulfil work tasks more effectively, to gain diversity in work tasks and to feel more satisfied and acknowledged. In this situation, mobility is driven by diverse and context-dependent individual interests, rather than by any systematic strategy of collective upward social mobility as described for classic professional projects (Larson, 1977).

Second, the opportunities for more self-determined and flexible work conditions were important 'drivers' for career moves, in particular the wished-for moves in the employees' own organisations. Autonomy and independence are highly individualised concepts that are connected with new hybrid forms and less hierarchical patterns of professional governance in organisations. In particular, the employees who moved from public health institutions, like hospitals, to a job at a spa perceived their new work as more flexible and independent. Self-determination, social benefits and the possibility of coordinating different spheres of their lives were important criteria underpinning their choice. However, contrary to the concept of entreployee, which suggests the increasing significance of work and market demands over the world of life, participants in the study put greater emphasis on convenience in the non-work sphere, including in family relationships. Consequently, the work/life balance and the relationship between autonomy and control must be assessed in the context of the social, cultural and economic conditions of the specific occupational field.

Third, there are nonetheless signs of an emerging occupational professionalism (Evetts, 2006) within the HWT sector, although developments are uneven. Professionalisation is low overall and limits the career possibilities of employees in this sector, but, at the same time, we observed higher levels of occupational control over work and more flexibility and autonomy for employees. In addition, self-governing practices of individuals are gaining significance in a situation where hierarchical governance practices are in the process of change towards more hybrid forms, and user demands – in our case, from guests – increasingly shape the work and associated tasks. Within this context of organisational and user demands and individual interests, a discourse of professionalism may serve the interests of different players and govern individuals effectively 'at a distance'. Furthermore, professional associations are still developing their roles, not least by establishing a monitoring system for professional education. These efforts are harbingers of a formalised knowledge system that is a key condition of professional power (Larson, 1977; Freidson, 1986, 2001; Abbott, 1988).

In the Hungarian spas the line between professionals and employees is still fluid, but the health and wellness-related occupational fields are eager to identify themselves as professions. HWT employees are gaining some recognition from service users and creating their own norms, sanctions and codes of ethics; they are in the process of 'embodying' the idea of being a professional in an emerging new field. This field shares some of the familiar tactics of the professions related to developments in the health sector, but it also encompasses new specific strategies of trans-sectoral mobility and individualised career paths. The HWT sector is therefore yet another variety of a professional project that is still in a state of flux.

References

Abbott, A. (1988) *The system of professions*, Chicago, IL: Chicago University Press.

Auster, C. (1996) *The sociology of work*, Thousand Oaks, CA: Pine Forge Press.

Collin, A. (1986) 'Career development: the significance of the subjective career', *Personnel Review*, vol 15, no 2, pp 22-8.

Evetts, J. (2003a) 'The sociological analysis of professionalism', *International Sociology*, vol 18, no 2, pp 395-415.

Evetts, J. (2003b) 'The sociology of professional groups: new questions and different explanations', *Knowledge, Work and Society*, vol 1, no 1, pp 33-56.

Evetts, J. (2006) 'The sociology of professional groups: new directions', *Current Sociology*, vol 54, no 1, pp 133-43.

Freidson, E. (1986) *Professional powers: A study of formal knowledge*, Chicago, IL: University of Chicago Press.

Freidson, E. (2001) *Professionalism: The third logic*, Oxford: Polity Press.

Gattiker, U. and Larwood, L. (1988) 'Predictors for managers' career mobility, success and satisfaction', *Human Relations*, vol 41, no 8, pp 569-91.

Guerrier, Y. (1987) 'Hotel managers' careers and their impact on hotels in Britain', *International Journal of Hospitality Management*, vol 6, no 3, pp 121-30.

Hall, R. (1994) *Sociology of work*, London: Pine Forge Press.

Hanlon, G. (1998) 'Professionalism as enterprise: service class politics and the redefinition of professionalism', *Sociology*, vol 32, no 1, pp 43-63.

Henninger, A. (2003) 'Der Arbeitskraftunternehmer und seine Frauen: Eine geschlechterkritische Revision des Analysekonzepts', in E. Kuhlmann and S. Betzelt (eds) *Geschlechterverhältnisse im Dienstleistungssektor*, Baden-Baden: Nomos, pp 119-32.

Hughes, E. (1958) *Men and their work*, New York: Free Press.

Kuhlmann, E. (2004) 'Post-modern times for professions: the fall of the "ideal professional" and its challenges to theory', *Knowledge, Work and Society*, vol 2, no 2, pp 69-89.

Ladkin, A. and Riley, M. (1994) 'Career theory and tourism: the development of a basic analytical framework', *Progress in Tourism and Hospitality Management*, vol 6, pp 225-37.

Ladkin, A. and Riley, M. (1996) 'Mobility and structure in the career paths of hotel managers: a labour market hybrid of the bureaucratic model?', *Tourism Management*, vol 17, no 6, pp 443-52.

Ladkin, A., Riley, M. and Szivas, E. (2002) *Tourism employment*, Clevedon: Channel View Publications.

Larson, M.S. (1977) *The rise of professionalism*, Berkeley, CA: University of California Press.

Montagna, P. (1977) *Occupations and society*, New Jersey, NJ: John Wiley.

Saks, M. (2003) 'The limitations of the Anglo-American sociology of the professions: a critique of the current dominant neo-Weberian orthodoxy', *Knowledge, Work and Society*, vol 1, no 1, pp 11-31.

Schein, E. (1971) 'The individual, the organization and the career: a conceptual scheme', *Journal of Applied Behavioural Science*, vol 7, pp 401-26.

Schein, E. (1984) 'Culture as an environmental context for careers', *Journal of Occupational Behaviour*, vol 5, no 1, pp 71-81.

Strauss, A.L. (2001) *Professions, work and careers*, New Brunswick, NJ: Transaction Publishers.

Van Maanen, J. and Schein, E. (1977) 'Improving the quality of work life: career development', in J. Hackman and J. Suttle (eds) *Improving life at work*, Santa Monica, CA: Goodyear.

Voß, G.G. and Pongratz, H.J. (1998) 'Der Arbeitskraftunternehmer', *Kölner Zeitschrift für Soziologie und Sozialpsychologie*, vol 50, no 1, pp 131-58.

Voß, G.G. and Pongratz, H.J. (2001) 'From employee to "entreployee" – towards a "self-entrepreneurial" work force?', *Concepts of Transformation*, vol 8, no 3, pp 239-54.

Watson, T. (1995) *Sociology of work and industry*, London: Routledge.

THIRTEEN

Migration and occupational integration: foreign health professionals in Portugal[1]

Joana Sousa Ribeiro

Introduction

Cross-border healthcare provision is being established as one of the policies of the European Union (EU). The free movement of goods, services and people – both patients and healthcare professionals – reflects the establishment of a single European market. The migration of healthcare workers is increasingly relevant in the provision of healthcare (Buchan, 2006). Although the EU aims to promote mobility, a number of structural and cultural barriers persist that impede the integration of foreign health professionals.

This chapter explores the obstacles to the mobility of healthcare professionals that exist in Portugal. The focus is on the existence of both formal and informal barriers to the professional mobility of doctors and nurses, taking different factors into account: the formal recognition of professional status, the process of socialisation and the negotiation of a professional identity in a culturally different workplace. The empirical material is taken from an ongoing qualitative research project with foreign nurses and doctors – from Spain and from outside the EU (the Republic of Moldavia, the Russian Federation, Ukraine and Romania, which at the time of the study had not joined the EU).

I argue that the healthcare sector creates a number of specific barriers to mobility and integration. Although the Bologna agreements harmonise the training system, country-specific competencies continue to matter. For instance, culture shapes the very concepts of disease, patient autonomy, confidentiality and multidisciplinary teamwork (Adel et al, 2004; Nicholas, 2006). It also shapes informal acknowledgement of diplomas and thus impacts on the level of trust that patients and colleagues put in foreign professionals. In addition, national regulation and regional policies have to be taken into account, such as shortage of doctors and long waiting lists for treatment in some countries. The examples highlight that the integration of foreign health professionals remains fundamentally an issue of the nation state and its cultural context. At the same time, however, the process of EU enlargement is producing its own dynamics.

The chapter starts with an overview of the debate on the migration of healthcare professionals. This is followed by statistical data on foreign human resources in the Portuguese National Health Service (NHS) – framing the macro level of the analysis – and micro-level analysis based on the findings from biographical interviews with physicians and nurses. Finally, some conclusions are drawn regarding barriers to integration and opportunity structures for foreign healthcare workers.

Migration of nurses and doctors: challenges to professional governance and integration

Foreign professionals place new challenges on the governance of healthcare, particularly on professional self-regulation. Differences in licensing and training programmes as well as professional tasks and boundaries reinforce an overall need for standardisation and assessment in order to 'protect patients' and to make professionals more accountable. New demands on professional governance are fundamentally the business of nation states and national professional associations. However, the emergence of a supranational legal framework for credentialing, as set out in EU Directives, stretches beyond national borders. Evetts (2006) argues that a common interpretation of the 'codes of conduct' is a prerequisite to the internationalisation of the professions (see also Jefferies and Evetts, 2000). As a consequence, the regulatory frameworks that shape the processes of professionalisation have diversified, not only in scope but also with respect to the interests of different groups involved in these processes.

The notion of interest-driven strategies involved in professionalisation processes points to a need for further differentiation between, within and across the two professional groups studied here. One particular challenge posed by migration is its intersection with other lines of division in the professional healthcare labour market, such as gender and age (Zulauf, 2001; see also Riska and Novelskaite, this volume). For instance, recent research highlights that marketisation and the logic of rationalisation create new social inequalities in professional projects with high proportions of women (Bourgeault, 2005; Henriksson et al, 2006). Gender remains relevant in the study of professions not only to the so-called female professions, but also to an increasingly sex-balanced medical profession.

Apart from the 'gendered-segregated character of the medical work' (Riska, 2001, p 184), female migrants have to overcome a number of invisible barriers – even prior to accreditation. The recognition of foreign qualifications is embedded in a framework that privileges men and 'masculine' occupations (Raghuram, 2004; Iredale, 2005). Furthermore, a gender bias is reinforced in the group of older immigrants seeking to re-establish themselves in the profession. Thus, governmental training programmes are especially relevant for those in a disadvantageous position in the occupation sphere – female and older professionals (Bernstein, 2000; Lerner and Menaheim, 2003).

Several authors point to the strategic significance of 'credentialing' and 'recredentialisation' in the integration process of healthcare migrants (Basran and Li, 1998; Lerner and Menaheim, 2003). Following Shuval (1998, p 309), credentialing is 'a political process in which the discourse reflects various groups' competitions for strategic control over jurisdiction and autonomy'. The concepts of 'credentialing' and 'jurisdiction' provide interesting links with theoretical approaches from the sociology of professions. For instance, Freidson (1994) explored the importance of licensing mechanisms in the definition of professional boundaries and the control of entry into a profession, and Abbott (1988) introduced the concept of 'jurisdiction' to explore negotiations and even 'professional wars' in a system of professions. From this perspective, the integration of foreign healthcare workers appears as yet another dimension of professional strategies in the interface between exclusionary tactics and social inclusion (Larson, 1977; Parkin, 1979; Saks and Kuhlmann, 2006). However, cultural differences in inter-occupational control may produce new ways of re-regulating the division of labour that need further empirical investigation. No data yet exist that provide convincing answers (Buchan, 2006), but recent research, mainly conducted in Anglo-American contexts, points to highly complex conditions of migration and professional integration (for instance, Zulauf, 2001; Buchan, 2002; Hawthorne, 2002; Raghuram and Kofman, 2002; Turrittin et al, 2002; Allan and Larsen, 2003; Ball, 2004; Yeates, 2004).

I argue that formal professional integration, based on a process of accreditation, is only one dimension of successful integration. A more complex 'map' of integration needs to be explored, one that includes social, cultural, political and symbolic dimensions – all of which shape the professional identity of the migrants (see also Shuval, 2000). As a consequence, the research links the macro- and meso-level analysis of the facilitators and structural barriers to micro-level analysis of professional trajectories, strategic actions and identity.

Foreign human resources in Portugal's National Health Service

The Portuguese healthcare system is a hybrid model of public and private financing and provision of healthcare services. Starting in 1979, the NHS established principles of centralised control, together with decentralised management. The Ministry of Health is the main provider and purchaser of care and is responsible for planning and management, although regulatory bodies operate at central and regional levels. In accordance with Portugal's Constitution, the NHS is mainly financed by general taxation and aims to provide universal coverage and nearly free access at the point of entry. However, inequalities persist due to a number of system deficits, such as the uneven geographical distribution of medical specialties, high levels of out-of-pocket payments and the introduction of user charges for inpatient care. In addition, the NHS in Portugal does not cover all healthcare needs – for instance adult dental care is excluded and has to be covered by private healthcare services.

More recently, and in line with international developments, internal markets and managerial principles have been introduced, but the impact on the quality of care is not yet clear. Although policy developments may challenge self-governing professional bodies, this is not a major policy goal in Portugal. The state–professions relationship in the Portuguese NHS seems to resemble what Burau and Vrangbæk (this volume) describe in the Italian system as 'complementary' and hybrid forms of governance, rather than the models of professional governance in the Anglo-Saxon NHS systems.

In Portugal doctors and nurses belong to self-regulatory professions, with each group having its own professional body that is responsible for professional ethics, accreditation and licensing, and, in cooperation with the Ministry of Health, the certification of specialist training. Consequently, professional self-regulatory bodies play a key role in the formal recognition of foreign-trained professionals and their integration in the national health workforce. The state–professions licensing process in particular provides a number of opportunities for informal facilitators or barriers to be established in the integration process. It is less clear, however, whether and how national professional bodies utilise these opportunities as 'boundary work' and demarcation strategies against their foreign colleagues.

Statistical data provide some information on workforce development with respect to foreign healthcare professionals in NHS institutions; only staff under the management of the Ministry of Health are included in the analysis as there are no data on private institutions (Table 13.1). From 1998 to 2003, the number of foreign health workers more than tripled, although NHS workers increased only slightly. In 2003 – our reference year when the interview data were gathered – the incidence of foreign workers among the total number of NHS staff was approximately 33 per 1,000. Seven per cent of physicians and 5% of nurses came

Table 13.1: Foreign human resources on the NHS staff, 1994–2003

Year	NHS professionals (total)	Foreign professionals	Incidence of foreign health professionals (1/1,000)
1994	104,585	313	2.99
1998	115,514	1,231	10.66
1999	115,464	2,150	18.62
2000	119,634	2,909	24.32
2001	122,236	3,374	27.60
2002	120,980	3,832	31.67
2003	123,962	4,069	32.82

Sources: 1994–2001: Ministry of Health, Department of Human Resources (2003); 2002–03: unpublished data, personal communication to the author, Ministry of Health, Department of Human Resources (2005)

from a foreign country; the latter is equivalent to the percentage of foreign workers in the Portuguese labour market as a whole (SOPEMI, 2004).

The Eastern European professionals are not yet statistically visible. However, their qualifications are increasingly recognised and they are an emerging group. Indeed, some studies showed the skilled scope of the Eastern European migration to Portugal and the overqualification for the jobs performed (Baganha et al, 2004).

Corresponding to the high proportion of female employees in the NHS, women also make up the majority of foreign professionals in both groups – some 60% (Ministry of Health, 2004). Physicians and nurses also represent 90% of the total foreign human resources working in the health sector. It is important to note that over half of the foreign female professionals in the health sector come from Spain. The Ravenstein law (Ravenstein, 1885), portraying women as more prone to migrate than men when short distances are involved, seems to apply to foreign professionals working in the Portuguese NHS.

Furthermore, foreign doctors and nurses in the NHS are younger than average. This result confirms behaviourist migration models that suggest a stronger tendency to migration among young adults and, as such, reflects the lifecourse. This tendency is especially true for nurses. However, on average foreign doctors are also younger than the average age of medical staff in Portugal, the majority of whom lie in the 35- to 40-year-old group.

In relation to the distribution of qualifications in the group of foreign doctors, the number of specialists and those in training programmes (for complementary and general internship) is broadly similar (see Figure 13.1).

Figure 13.1: Foreign physicians by occupational status, 2003

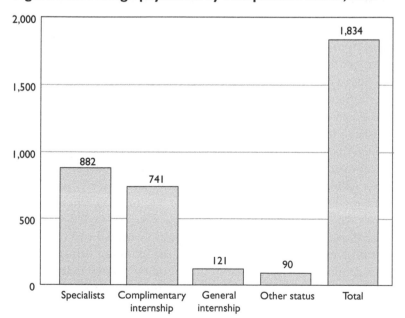

Source: Ministry of Health, Department of Human Resources

The situation is different in nursing. Here, foreign nurses began their career in Portugal mainly as first-level nurses, that is to say, at the bottom of the workforce (Table 13.2). As the nurses are, on average, very young (under 31 years old), few of them have the competencies necessary for higher-status positions in the nursing profession.

Table 13.2: Foreign nurses by professional status and gender, 2003

Professional status	Women	Men	Total
Nurse	1,341	562	1,903
Chief nurse	4	1	5
Specialist nurse	10	1	11
Graduated nurse	30	9	39
Supervisor nurse	4	2	6
Professor	2	0	2
Total	1,391	575	1,966

Source: College of Nurses (2004), personal communication to the author, unpublished data

We can conclude that the two professional groups differ with respect to some demographic characteristics, such as age, gender and occupational status, which are likely to impact on processes of integration. Qualitative analysis further highlights how these factors impact on and intersect with other positions.

Integration of foreign health professionals – snakes and ladders

Migrant workers from Spain and non-EU countries have different positions, not only with respect to formal licensing procedures, but also regarding culture, language and identity. This section presents the findings from two case studies, one comprising EU migrants and the second Eastern European, non-EU migrants.

The analysis is based on 58 biographical interviews, conducted with Spanish, Moldavian, Russian and Ukrainian nurses and doctors in 2003, selected from a database of their first enrolment in a qualifications recognition programme. Additionally, semi-structured interviews were conducted with institutional actors, such as the Ministry of Health, physicians' association, nurses' association, and nursing and medical schools. The interviews focused on three areas of integration. First, access to employment, in particular acknowledgement of diplomas and recruitment processes; second, integration related to professional status, collaboration within the working team, and the existence of institutional discrimination; and third, career progression measured by acknowledgement of specialisation and participation in advanced training programmes.

Case study 1: Intra-European mobility and integration of health professionals

Both nurses and doctors from Spain, faced with a saturated healthcare labour market at home, chose Portugal for its labour market opportunities. The Portuguese educational system is a further important variable when analysing the push-pull factors. With regard to nurses, Portugal offers four-year graduation courses, instead of three years in Spain. However, Spanish nurses' access to these courses is restricted. First, the process of formal recognition of their Spanish diplomas for academic purposes is time-consuming. Second, the institutions responsible for their graduation give priority to Portugal's own students. Doctors, by contrast, benefit from the training opportunities in the Portuguese system, as access to specialist training is easier than in Spain. The majority of doctors moved to Portugal for postgraduate education, in order to specialise. The Spanish system involves taking an extremely difficult examination as a precondition of specialist training, the MIR, based on a year of full-time preparation without any financial reward.

Until recently, therefore, barriers to specialist training were lower in Portugal than in Spain. However, the tide is turning, and a number of formal and informal procedures are gaining ground in Portugal. On top of this, the Portuguese physicians' association changed the rules of access to specialisation. Since 2006, all doctors have to undertake an internship, which is included in the first year of the specialist training. Furthermore, entitlement to specialty training prescribes not only the recognition of diplomas, but also theoretical and communication examinations. The communication examination was introduced in 1998 for all applicants, precisely when the number of Spanish professionals working in Portugal was on the increase. Since August 2006, this examination is only compulsory for students from non-Portuguese-speaking universities, thus hindering the integration of Spanish doctors. Added to this, the interviews highlight a number of obstacles in collecting the necessary information on labour market and licensing requirements; even the physicians' association does not provide reliable information. In this situation, professional networks are crucial in order to establish a 'migration chain', bypassing information barriers.

The various barriers to integration not only challenge the professionals and hinder their individual integration and career opportunities. Numerous practices of discrimination – and even precarious work situations – also challenge the safety of patients and the governance of professional performance, including malpractice (Abbing, 1997; De Bijl and van de Kragt, 1997). For instance, some nurses have started working in public hospitals without a professional licence. While this may be a temporary problem caused by a delay in the recognition of their diplomas, some types of labour market contracts pose serious risks to the quality of care and the safety of patients, as the following examples highlight.

Some Spanish doctors living close to the border work in accident and emergency departments of hospitals in both countries. This double employment can entail working a 48-hour shift for emergency care. Consequently, the precarious 'lump sum contracts' of doctors may be a serious risk to quality of care. Another example of precarious contracts, although not as risky for patients and mainly reported in the group of nurses, are short-term contracts of three or six months that provide too little opportunity for integration in the organisation of healthcare in a culturally different workplace. A third form of precarious contract and discrimination was reported by the group of doctors. Some doctors are obliged to work in more than one health centre, which invariably leads to overtime. This mainly happens in areas with a shortage of doctors – like paediatrics and public health – if their specialisation is not or not yet recognised. The interviews revealed a number of difficulties in the process of recognition of specialisation: for example, a female paediatrician who is working as a general practitioner (GP) and planning a second specialisation in Portugal stated: 'We arrive here with a certificate [the Portuguese School of Medicine] according a minimum passing grade [this makes it] very difficult to compete with your peers who did their exam here' (MM3).

One major problem is recognition of the qualification in professional, but not in academic, terms. This may explain why Spanish doctors work more often in specialties that are 'second choice' for Portuguese doctors – such as anaesthesiology, family medicine or internal medicine. However, it is interesting to note that these 'second choice' specialties do not necessarily overlap with a gendered segregation of specialties, and are not fully in line with international findings (see, for instance, Riska, 2001). Instead, these foreign qualified professionals reproduce a nation-specific pattern of gendered specialties in the medical profession in Portugal: women doctors more often work in paediatrics, gynaecology, dermatology, clinic pathology and internal medicine (Ribeiro, 2004).

Occupational segregation is also observed in the nursing profession, but here it is mainly an issue of the tasks involved and their position in the occupational hierarchy. One important factor is age. As previously mentioned, Spanish nurses are on average very young and consequently started a career in Portugal as first-level nurses. Another problem arises from the differences in the occupational structure and the tasks of nurses in the two health systems. In Spain the health occupational structure is more diversified and nurses habitually delegate tasks to nursing assistants, while nurses in the Portuguese system often also provide basic care, such as washing patients. This nation-specific structure of the nursing workforce together with the age composition of the Spanish nurses may therefore reinforce the perception of downgrading of professional competencies and loss of autonomy in this group.

The structural and demographic factors hindering the process of integration often intersect with individual perceptions and cultural factors. For instance, a lack of language abilities together with the absence of any communication exam for nurses nurtures an overall mistrust in language competencies that, in turn, impacts on the individual perceptions of the foreign qualified professionals and limits their scope of action. As a consequence, foreign nurses often work in units where communication with patients is less important, such as in theatre or intensive care.

Apart from language problems, a number of tensions arise from the presence of the Spanish nurses in the teams. One area of conflict is greater instability in working hours. According to a Portuguese nursing director, the Spanish nurses try to exchange rotas with their compatriots if they can, in order to make short visits to Spain possible. Further conflicts may arise from cultural differences in the regulation of professional conduct and workforce relationships. Another area of conflict is the attitudes of patients, which may even be perceived as discrimination. As one nurse reported: 'They didn't want to be assisted by a Spanish nurse. It was quite evident, but nobody came out and said it directly' (EN3).

Case study 2: Integration of non-EU health professionals

Physicians and nurses coming to Portugal from (at the time of the study) non-EU Eastern European countries are faced with the devaluation of their competencies at the first stage of migration. They enter the unskilled and low-status labour market; the men as bricklayers or machine operators, the women as maids or employees in restaurants, bakeries and poultry farms. The interviews highlighted that the experience of occupational and social downgrading is perceived as a serious threat to their professional identity and challenges professional migrants in various ways.

Women may have better opportunities than men, especially nurses. They search for a job more actively, contacting health institutions; and they more often work in the allied healthcare professions. Here, although they find themselves demoted to a low-status position, they have the opportunity to learn about the Portuguese healthcare system, the organisation of care and the medical language, thereby improving cultural integration in the organisation as well as language and country-specific communication skills. However, downgrading of professional status may also lead to frustration and negatively affect their commitment to the job or 'job involvement', defined by Kanungo (1982, p 342) as a 'belief descriptive of the present job ... [which] tends to be a function of how much the job can satisfy one's present needs'. A statement from a Moldavian migrant working as a nursing assistant points in a similar direction: 'I go to the hospitals, I see lots of patients, many cases. I see, but I have no right to do anything ... I don't even have the right to put in an intravenous drip' (LN7).

The recruitment of foreign professionals for low-skilled caring occupations is a strategy to substitute higher skills for lower expenses; unsurprisingly, the foreign professionals perceived this strategy as discrimination.

Apart from individuals' efforts to improve their labour market position, the process of licensing and foreign diploma recognition is vital in gaining access to a high-skilled healthcare labour market. Here, medical and nursing schools act as gatekeepers. Recognition involves a training period for both professional groups, and additional exams for physicians (see case study 1). After passing exams, nurses and doctors have the right to register with the corresponding associations. Portuguese law prescribes that registration takes place within three months, but the difficulty of obtaining the required documents from their native countries often causes delays of up to six months. The process of licensing is thus time-consuming, bureaucratic and expensive – 6,000 euros in the case of doctors – and not compatible with a full-time job.

To facilitate this process, most of the foreign professionals in our case study were enrolled in a programme. This programme is financially supported by a foundation and EU funds and managed by a non-governmental organisation, and its aim is to advance the recognition of diplomas in medicine (since 2002) and nursing studies (since 2005) for workers from countries for which there is no automatic recognition of qualifications. Financial support was granted to the participants in the programme immediately after they started training.

The applicants were mainly advised to enrol in this programme through Portuguese social networks. However, all participants stated that they also needed support from and relied on social networks – mainly female family members – in their country of origin. The role of networks in the process of licensing highlights the significance of social integration in their home country as well as in Portugal. The training period was particularly problematic for older physicians, as they had to balance the lack of professional recognition and their physical appearance in a gendered and age-discriminating labour market. A Moldavian male physician reported: 'It happened in paediatrics, where the female physician was slim and I am big. Everybody looked at me. Because at my age, you're a doctor, not a student. And that bothers me a little' (LP10).

However, the findings indicate that older male doctors were more successful at blending in with their Portuguese peers, while older female doctors faced more difficulties in affirming and upholding their professional identity. In this respect, the research in Portugal mirrors the results of other studies (Lerner and Menaheim, 2003).

As in the group of Spanish migrants, informal discrimination and cultural differences also impact and may reinforce institutional barriers. However, although areas of conflict sometimes overlap, there are also important differences here. For instance, participants in this study reported discrimination on the part of Portuguese tutors. At the same time, there are also specific sources of support for the migrants from outside the EU. For example, doctors received support from the PALOP – the Portuguese-speaking African countries – in particular during the examination for the credential recognition, and from Spanish professionals during the training period. In contrast to doctors, however, Spanish nurses did not welcome their colleagues from Eastern European countries. One reason for the lack of support in the group of nurses may be greater competition: the programme for foreign nurses started in 2005, when labour market opportunities started to fall.

However, these explanations are not fully convincing. Moreover, the differences between the two occupational groups point to greater professional cohesion and solidarity in the medical profession, which – following classical patterns – acts more collectively. The picture of a profession standing shoulder to shoulder starts to disintegrate, however, when foreign doctors pass the examination and enter the labour market.

As observed in the group of Spanish migrants, both doctors and nurses were more often found in professional segments with lower prestige, such as health centres (doctors) and community care services (nurses). Furthermore, doctors often worked as GPs because their specialisation was not recognised. For example, a Russian female neonatologist was recruited by a public hospital with private management as a GP, but worked as a specialist providing paediatric services. The same happens with nurses who specialised in obstetrics: they are employed as general nurses, but provide obstetric and gynaecological services.

In both professional groups we see a mismatch between the labour contract and the actual tasks performed; occupational downgrading and discrimination therefore seem to be very strong in the group of Eastern European migrants. At the same time, it is precisely these areas of the healthcare sector that provide an opportunity for political integration. These areas are considered essential to the Portuguese health system and may thus facilitate the acquisition of residents' permits, making visas redundant. Consequently, the political integration of these professional groups is closely linked to, and depends on, the success of their professional integration in the health workforce.

Conclusion

This chapter has explored the processes of integration of foreign professionals in healthcare systems, taking the Portuguese NHS as an example. Although mobility of human resources is an increasingly important policy goal in the EU, there is a significant gap between supranational policies and national opportunity structures for successful integration. The research highlights the persistence of a number of serious barriers to the integration of foreign doctors and nurses in Portugal.

One conclusion to be drawn from the findings is the need to assess the processes and connectedness of different mechanisms that form the specific pathways of integration. These pathways include cultural integration, like knowledge of Portuguese language; political integration, for instance knowledge of European Directives and how to obtain permission for residency; social integration, networks in particular but also participation in specific programmes; and symbolic and institutional integration, especially formal recognition of diplomas. In both professional groups, and regardless of the country of graduation, integration depends on relationships between a multitude of different actors. Apart from the role of national governments in the regulation of welfare professions and migration policies, private employers, foundations, non-governmental organisations, supranational entities (like the European Court of Justice) and national professional bodies shape the practices of formal and informal recognition and may either further or hinder the integration of foreign professionals. Furthermore, more informal factors, in particular the attitudes of patients and colleagues, are highly relevant in the processes of integrating foreign workers in the organisation of care.

Even within the EU we conclude that professional qualifications – for instance, medical specialisation – are difficult to transfer from one country to another. Although the EU supports a European market in people and goods, the mobility of professionals does not easily fit with the conditions and interests of national regulatory frameworks, including the self-regulatory bodies of doctors and nurses. A number of formal procedures and informal mechanisms were identified as barriers, including slow and difficult licensing procedures, precarious working conditions and even overt discrimination. Accordingly, the interests of both the healthcare organisations and the professions may counteract the enlargement of career options and mobility and, more generally, the emergence of a de facto union of Europe.

A further conclusion relates to the comparison between the occupational mobility of professionals from within the EU (Spain) and non-EU countries in Eastern Europe. The findings draw attention to barriers to integration, some of which point to greater difficulties for foreign health professionals from non-EU countries. Greater difficulties in the licensing process and labour market integration, for example, cause more serious experiences of downgrading and discrimination than in the group of Spanish migrants. The comparison underscores that, even in times of globalisation and supranational policies, the national and local institutional arrangements and cultural conditions do not lose their significance.

Finally, the findings raise a number of classic issues in the study of professions, such as the different configurations of professional interests and the mechanisms of occupational closure, as well as the role of the state (Larson, 1977; Johnson et al, 1995). However, bringing migration and mobility into the equation makes the state–professions relationship and the definition of professional and public interests even more complex and puts new issues on the agenda. One novel insight is that the market interests of national professional players seem to be a stronger force than a collective cross-border, professional identity. 'Boundary work' and strategies of exclusion increasingly take place within a profession and the self-regulatory professional bodies are mainly a source of power for national professional players. Foreign health professionals not only place new demands on professional governance and occupational integration, they also challenge the concept of both the 'private interest government of professions' and the 'public interest'.

Note
[1] This chapter draws on a PhD thesis, supervised by Professor Maria Ioannis Baganha and financially supported by the Science and Technology Foundation,

Portuguese Science and the Technology Ministry. I would also like to thank Maria Ioannis Baganha and the editors for their helpful comments.

References

Abbing, R. (1997) 'The right of the patient to quality of medical practice and the position of migrant doctors within the EU', *European Journal of Health Law*, vol 4, pp 347-60.

Abbott, A. (1988) *The system of professions: An essay on the division of expert labour*, Chicago, IL: University of Chicago Press.

Adel, M., Blau, W., Dobson, J., Hoesh, K. and Salt, J. (2004) 'Recruitment and the migration of foreign workers in health and social care', *IMIS-Beiträge*, no 25, pp 201-30.

Allan, H. and Larsen, A. (2003) *We need respect: Experience of internationally recruited nurses in the UK*, London: Royal College of Nursing.

Baganha, I., Marques, J. and Góis, P. (2004) 'Novas Migrações, Novos Desafios: a imigração do leste europeu', *Revista Crítica de Ciências Sociais*, no 69, pp 95-115.

Ball, R.E. (2004) 'Divergent development, racialised rights: globalised labour markets and the trade of nurses – the case of the Philippines', *Women's Studies International Forum*, vol 27, no 2, pp 119-33.

Basran, G. and Li, Z. (1998) 'Devaluation of foreign credentials as perceived by visible minority professional immigrants', *Canadian Ethnic Studies*, vol 30, no 3, pp 7-23.

Bernstein, J. (2000) 'The professional self-evaluation of immigrant physicians from the former Soviet Union in Israel', *Journal of Immigrant Health*, vol 2, no 4, pp 183-90.

Bourgeault, I. (2005) 'Rationalization of health care and female professional projects: reconceptualizing the role of medicine, the state and health care institutions from a gendered perspective', *Knowledge, Work and Society*, vol 3, no 1, pp 27-52.

Buchan, J. (2002) *International recruitment of nurses: UK case study*, London: World Health Organization, International Council of Nurses and Royal College of Nursing.

Buchan, J. (2006) 'Migration of health workers in Europe: policy problem or policy solution?', in C.-A. Dubois, M. McKee and E. Nolte (eds) *Human resources for health in Europe*, European Observatory on Health Systems and Policies Series, Milton Keynes: Open University Press, pp 66-87.

De Bijl, N. and van de Kragt, I.N. (1997) 'Legal safeguards against medical practice by not suitably qualified persons: a comparative study in seven EU-countries', *European Journal of Health Law*, vol 4, no 1, pp 5-18.

Evetts, J. (2006) 'Global and local professionalism: centralised regulation or occupational trust', Paper presented to the European Sociological Association Interim Conference, Research Network 'Sociology of Professions', Bremen, Germany, 30 March-1 April.

Freidson, E. (1994) *Professionalism reborn: Theory, prophecy and policy*, Cambridge: Polity Press.

Hawthorne, L. (2002) 'Qualifications recognition reform for skilled migrants in Australia: applying competency-based assessment to overseas-qualified nurses', *International Migration Review*, vol 40, no 6, pp 55-92.

Henriksson, L., Wrede, S. and Burau, V. (2006) 'Understanding professional projects in welfare service work: revival of old professionalism?', *Gender, Work and Organization*, vol 13, no 2, pp 174-92.

Iredale, R. (2005) 'Gender, immigration policies and accreditation: valuing the skills of professional women migrants', *Geoforum*, vol 36, no 2, pp 155-66.

Jefferies, D. and Evetts, J. (2000) 'Approaches to the international recognition of professional qualifications in engineering and the sciences', *European Journal of Engineering Education*, vol 25, no 1, pp 99-107.

Johnson, T., Larkin, G. and Saks, M. (eds) (1995) *Health professions and the state in Europe*, London: Routledge.

Kanungo, R. (1982) 'Measurement of job and work involvement', *Journal of Applied Psychology*, vol 67, no 3, pp 341-9.

Larson, M. (1977) *The rise of professionalism: A sociological analysis*, Berkeley, CA: University of California Press.

Lerner, M. and Menaheim, G. (2003) 'Decredentialization and recredentialization', *Work and Occupations*, vol 30, no 1, pp 3-29.

Ministry of Health, Department of Human Resources (2003) *Recursos Humanos Estrangeirous – 2001*, Lisboa: DMRS.

Ministry of Health, Department of Human Resources (2004) Statistics, www.dmrs.min-saude.pt/recursos_dados_estatisticos_4.asp

Nicholas, S. (2006) 'The challenges of the free movement of health professionals', in M. McKee, L. MacLehose and E. Nolte (eds) *Health policy and EU enlargement*, European Observatory on Health Systems and Policies Series, Milton Keynes: Open University Press, pp 97-122.

Parkin, F. (1979) *Marxism and class theory: A bourgeois critique*, London: Tavistock.

Raghuram, P. (2004) 'The difference that skills make: gender, family migration strategies and regulated labour markets', *Journal of Ethnic and Migration Studies*, vol 30, no 2, pp 303-21.

Raghuram, P. and Kofman, E. (2002) 'State, labour markets and immigration: overseas doctors in the UK', *Environment and Planning A*, vol 34, no 11, pp 2071-89.

Ravenstein, E. (1885) 'The laws of migration', *Journal of Royal Statistical Society*, vol 48, no 2, pp 167-235.

Ribeiro, J.S. (2004) *Imigração Independente em Portugal: o caso dos profissionais qualificados no sector da saúde*, www.apdemografia.pt/pdf_Congresso/1_Joana_Sousa_Ribeiro.pdf

Riska, E. (2001) 'Towards gender balance: but will women physicians have an impact on medicine?', *Social Science and Medicine*, vol 52, pp 179-87.

Saks, M. and Kuhlmann, E. (2006) 'Introduction: professions, social inclusion and citizenship: challenge and change in European health systems', *Knowledge, Work and Society*, vol 4, no 1, pp 9-20.

Shuval, J. T. (1998) 'Some latent functions of credentialing: the case of immigrant physicians to Israel', in V. Olgiati, L. Orzack and M. Saks (eds) *Professions, identity and order in comparative perspective*, Onati: International Institute for the Sociology of Law, pp 307-22.

Shuval, J. T. (2000) 'The reconstruction of professional identity among immigrant physicians in three societies', *Journal of Immigrant Health*, vol 2, no 4, pp 191-202.

SOPEMI (2004) *Trends in international migration – 2003*, Paris: OECD.

Turrittin, J., Hagey, R., Guruge, S., Collins, E. and Mitchell, M. (2002) 'The experiences of professional nurses who have migrated to Canada: cosmopolitan citizenship or democratic racism?', *International Journal of Nursing Studies*, vol 39, no 6, pp 655-67.

Yeates, N. (2004) 'A dialogue with global care chain analysis: nurse migration in the Irish context', *Feminist Review*, no 77, pp 79-95.

Zulauf, M. (2001) *Migrant women – professionals in the European Union*, New York: Palgrave.

FOURTEEN

Professionals in transition: physicians' careers, migration and gender in Lithuania

Elianne Riska and Aurelija Novelskaite

Introduction

During recent decades, migration has become one of the most significant social forces influencing the labour market, and 'skilled migration is rapidly becoming one of the major components of migration streams in many parts of the world' (Raghuram, 2004, p 163; see also Guibernau and Rex, 1997). There are, however, few studies that focus on the migration of high-status professionals – for example, lawyers, scientists, physicians. The dearth of research on this group might be related to the assumed unproblematic character of this kind of migration. Migration of highly skilled professionals is welcomed and has been facilitated and encouraged by governments in developed countries. Migrating professionals 'have been absorbed into the labour market to such an extent that they become virtually invisible and are rarely the subject of public debate' (Ryan, 2005, p 384). Nevertheless, the scope and the directions of this kind of migration are worth exploring (see also Ribeiro, this volume). Studies indicate that the migration of highly skilled workers has a pattern quite different from that of unskilled workers (Guibernau and Rex, 1997). Hence, research on the migration of professionals may contribute significantly to both the sociology of professions and theories of international migration.

Research on transnational migration tends to examine migrating men and does not address the gender dynamics of this transnational process (Raghuram, 2004; Budani, 2005; Ryan, 2005). Studies that include women or focus on female emigrants' experiences tend to examine mainly family-related issues – for example, childcare and cultivation of ties with relatives left behind (Ryan, 2005) – rather than women's endeavours in the professions.

The past dominant neo-Weberian approach in research on professions has emphasised professional unity and professions as national professional projects (Leicht and Fennell, 2001). Evetts (1999) has noted that within-state theorising has therefore dominated sociological research on professions. Nevertheless, members of professions like medicine are increasingly internationally mobile, and both enlargement of and the harmonisation of regulations within the European Union (EU) have facilitated a free movement of professionals within the EU. Yet, most studies on the migration of physicians have looked at the mobility of physicians from developing countries – for example, Africa or Asia – to richer Western societies (for instance, Astor et al, 2005; Hagopian et al, 2005), and only a few have looked at the migration of women physicians (for instance, Harrison, 1998). Hence, there is a need to look from a gender perspective at the career mobility of physicians outside state boundaries.

This chapter explores how institutional arrangements have changed and created new opportunities and constraints for physicians in post-Soviet societies like Lithuania. It examines how professional mobility is shaped in post-Soviet societies and to what extent decisions to practise in the future in an EU country is related to gender.

The Lithuanian healthcare system in the post-Soviet era

The Republic of Lithuania is (like Estonia and Latvia) one of the Baltic countries. It is a small country both in area and in population (3.7 million people). The Lithuanian healthcare system experienced three national reforms during the 20th century. Between 1918 and 1940, the system developed along the Bismarck model (see Kuhlmann, this volume, on the German model); then when Lithuania was annexed to the Soviet Union after the Second World War, Soviet medicine (Field, 1957), or the Semashko model (Stevens, 2005), superseded the old model. Since 1990, when Lithuania regained its political and economical independence, the healthcare system has been under transformation with the aim of developing a three-level system, with general practitioners (GPs) at the first level.

In Soviet society the character of the medical profession changed in two respects. First, the profession lost its traditional professional status, because medical education was transferred to vocational schools, although not in Lithuania. Second, physicians became a group of state employees among other employees in the bureaucratic Soviet society. The profession lost its autonomy and thereby its control over the education and work of its members. Meanwhile, the physician's work became women's work: in 1950, 77% of the physicians in the Soviet Union were women (Field, 1957, 1967; Ryan, 1989; Riska, 2001a). This historic example has been used to support the argument that when a profession loses status, it becomes female-dominated. The thesis about the 'feminisation' of a profession has therefore suggested a link between the numerical increase of women and a loss of status of the profession (Charles and Grusky, 2004; for a critical analysis see Riska, 2001b). Nevertheless, in the Soviet Union the low status of the health professions was related more to the high prestige and high salaries of the industrial (male) worker than to the gender composition of the health professions per se (Field, 1957, 1967; Ryan, 1989).

The fall of the Soviet Union resulted not only in a gradual marketisation of healthcare, but also in reprofessionalisation – that is, an effort to re-establish the academic and professional status of the medical profession (Field, 1991; Twigg, 2000; Rivkin-Fish, 2005). This endeavour has been more vibrant in those post-Soviet societies – like Estonia and Lithuania – that before the Second World War had a traditional medical profession trained along Western lines.

In March 1990 Lithuania declared its independence and embarked on a long journey to reform its economy and healthcare system. Today the system is organised in a hierarchical and integrated way: the Ministry of Health is responsible for tertiary care hospitals, while the local governments are responsible for the provision of about 60% of public health services, including polyclinics (about 150 across the country) and small hospitals (WHO, 1996). In 1991 Lithuania started to implement a statutory health insurance scheme, which was put into effect in 1997, and administered by the State Social Insurance Agency (WHO, 1996).

As Osinsky and Mueller (2004, p 195) in their study of professionals in Russia point out, two features of the post-Soviet period are different from the Anglo-American characteristics of the status of professionals. First, most professionals in the post-Soviet societies continue to work in the public sector and its institutions. Second, most professional practices are incorporated in the hierarchical structures of the state. Hence the conflict is not so much the interprofessional competition of jurisdiction in a market-based economy (Abbott, 1988) as the relation of the profession to the state (Jones, 1991). Freidson (2001) has pointed to the threats of bureaucratic organisations to the ideals inherent in professionalism and the work of professions. These conditions are also relevant for understanding the status of professions in the transitional stage in Lithuania.

The supply of physicians in Lithuania is one of the highest in Europe: in 1994 there were 4.0 doctors per 1,000 population (compared to 1.6 in the UK) and in 2000 the rate was still 3.8 (WHO, 1996, p 30; Gaižauskienė et al, 2002, p 10). About 90% of the physicians are employed in public hospitals and polyclinics on a salaried basis. The internal division of labour in the medical profession diversified after the possibilities of specialising were introduced. During the Soviet era, in Lithuania there was no special postgraduate training after basic medical education, and therefore a system of physician training in residencies was introduced in 1994 (Gaižauskienė et al, 2002).

In both Estonia and Lithuania the medical profession had become female-dominated during the Soviet era: in Estonia in 1991, 77% of physicians were women (Barr, 1995; Barr and Boyle, 2001); and in Lithuania in 2004, 70% of physicians were women (Table 14.1). The proportion of women physicians is expected to increase: women constituted 57% of first-year medical students at Kaunas University of Medicine in 1989, 65% in 1995 and 82% in 2001 (Gaižauskienė et al, 2002, pp 12-13).

Although women constitute a high proportion of physicians in Lithuania, women are not evenly distributed in medical specialties and hence are not represented in the same proportion as they are in the profession as a whole (Table 14.1). Women are well represented in specialties that confirm essentialist notions of women's tasks: child and adolescent psychiatry, geriatrics and paediatrics. Paediatrics is almost exclusively (93%) a women's specialty, while surgery is a markedly male-dominated field in Lithuania: women constitute only 11% of surgeons.

Table 14.1: Proportion of women physicians in selected medical specialties in Lithuania, 1998–2004

Specialty	% of women
Anaesthesiology	56
Child and adolescent psychiatry	85
General practice	85
Geriatrics	90
Internal medicine	79
Pathology	48
Paediatrics	93
Psychiatry	69
Obstetrics and gynaecology	76
Ophthalmology	88
General surgery	11
All physicians	70

Source: Ministry of Health of Republic of Lithuania (2000)

Recent public discourse on the emigration of Lithuanians focuses on particular social groups, for example scientists and physicians (Stankønienë, 1996). In the past, the intention to migrate was assessed in neutral or even positive terms, while the recent migration of professionals, like physicians, is viewed as a threat for Lithuania (Gliosaitë, 2004; Marcinkevičienë, 2004). A survey was conducted in 2002 among Lithuanian physicians and medical residents about their intentions of working in the EU in the future. The results showed that 61% of the residents and 26% of the physicians intended to leave for the EU or other countries (Stankunas et al, 2004). Fifteen per cent of the medical residents and 5% of the physicians planned to leave for good. Furthermore, there were gender differences in the intention to migrate: male residents, almost as often as female residents, reported that they planned to leave for the EU (62% and 59% respectively), while female physicians slightly more often than male physicians planned to leave for the EU (27% and 22% respectively) (Gaižauskienë et al, 2002).

This chapter examines the gendered attitudes on career options, market conditions and migration among Lithuanian physicians. Lithuania is used as a case study of a post-Soviet society in transition and a society in which women constitute a majority of the physicians (70%) and where, therefore, the intention of women physicians to migrate would not be a marginal phenomenon. In a 'feminised' profession like the one in Lithuania, how do the three determinants or 'logics' (Freidson, 2001) of the conditions of the medical profession – professional autonomy, the market and the bureaucracy of the state – influence decisions to stay or to leave the national medical profession and become part of a larger international community of professionals?

Methods and material

The data for this study were collected by means of a questionnaire and semi-structured interviews. There was no complete national register of physicians, as is available in Western countries, particularly a database that would provide information by gender (Gaižauskienė et al, 2002). A snowball sample was therefore considered a reliable method for collecting the data for this study.

A self-administered questionnaire was distributed to 137 pre-selected physicians (54 men and 83 women) in Kaunas and Vilnius between April and August of 2005: 65% practised in Kaunas; 31% were paediatricians, 17% were GPs, 15% were surgeons and 34% were from various other specialties (for detailed information on the composition of these groups, see the note to Table 14.2). The physicians worked in various types of settings: small private clinics, state polyclinics and hospitals, and university clinics. The stratified distribution of three specialties – paediatrics, general practice and surgery – was related to the broader inquiry on gender and medical practice (Table 14.1).

The questionnaire (in Lithuanian) explored four themes, each by means of seven items: professional commitment, career opportunity, external opportunities and collegiality. The responses were recorded on five-point Likert scales ranging from 1 (strongly disagree) to 5 (strongly agree). The questionnaire was adapted from a study on Russian professionals and state employees and their professional orientation and commitment (Osinsky and Mueller, 2004). Two items are used as indicators of attitudes towards international professional career mobility:

- *exit opportunity (EO)* consists of the statement 'I could leave for another country without any problems' and is one of the items that measure external opportunities;
- *international career opportunity (ICO)* consists of the statement 'I have very good opportunities to leave for foreign countries to develop my professional career' and is one of the statements that measure career opportunity.

The questionnaire data were analysed by SPSS 13.0 for Windows. In addition to descriptive statistical information about physicians' attitudes towards professional commitment, T-tests (and their non-parametric equivalent Mann–Whitney U tests when the groups under analysis were too small) were used in the examination of women's and men's responses. The method allows us to evaluate the statistical significance of the difference between the average evaluations of the two items. In reading the results it has to be remembered that they cannot be generalised to describe the whole population of Lithuanian physicians, because our study population was stratified and was therefore not statistically representative of all Lithuanian physicians.

The items in the questionnaire were illuminated further by semi-structured interviews. The interviews were conducted between April and June of 2005 among surgeons and paediatricians (*N*=36, 15 men and 21 women), who practised in Kaunas and Vilnius in Lithuania in 2005. These two medical specialties were selected in order to obtain representation of the gender proportions in these two specialties. A total of 21 paediatricians (14 women and 7 men) and 15 surgeons (8 men and 7 women) were interviewed.

The interview schedule contained 18 questions that mapped the choice of medicine as a vocation and specialty, professional identity, changes in medicine, gendered and cultural aspects of practice, career opportunities, migration and family. The interviews were conducted in Lithuanian and lasted on average between 40 and 60 minutes, and were tape-recorded and fully transcribed. All interviews were translated into English. Accounts of physicians' attitudes to the possibilities of emigrating and developing their career in a foreign country are drawn on in this chapter.

A grounded theory approach to the analysis of the qualitative data was used (Glaser and Strauss, 1967; Charmaz, 2006). After an initial reading of all the transcribed interviews a selection of key themes emerged. The analysis of the data proceeded by means of focused coding (Charmaz, 2006) and in the analysis of the data the coding frame 'migration' was used. Both researchers in this study read all the interviews and assessed the agreement on the coding frame.

Gendered attitudes towards the possibilities of emigration

Migration was not a major priority for the Lithuanian physicians. A third of the respondents feel they could leave for another country without any problems. Yet, half of the respondents do not think that that they would have good opportunities for a successful career in medicine in another country. There is a gender difference in the attitudes about the possibilities of migration: men are more positive than women both about these possibilities and about career opportunities abroad (Table 14.2). For example, 42% of the men think in positive terms about migrating and 29% in positive terms about career opportunities abroad, against 26% and 13% respectively of the women; the mean difference of the male and female physicians' evaluations of opportunities to develop a professional career abroad is statistically significant ($t=3,9$; $p<0,01$.) In fact, women are rather pessimistic about their career opportunities abroad: 63% of the female respondents do not believe that they could successfully practise medicine in a foreign country, while only 31% of the men think that.

There are marked differences between the specialty groups in their views on migrating. Paediatricians and GPs are least inclined to think they would leave Lithuania: only 23% of paediatricians and 21% of GPs, as compared to 38% of surgeons and 45% of physicians from mixed specialties, think they could leave the country without any problems. Furthermore, paediatricians are least inclined to think that they would have good opportunities to develop their career in a foreign country (9%), followed by GPs (13%), surgeons (19%) and other specialists (34%). When male and female physicians are analysed by specialty, the within-group differences show that paediatricians and GPs have considerably higher aspirations regarding a successful career in a foreign country than surgeons, but those who are in other specialties have the highest career ambitions (Table 14.2).

Surgeons believe on average that they have better career opportunities for practice abroad than do paediatricians and GPs. However, there are marked differences in the mean responses on this issue: men are more optimistic than women (men = 2.7 out of 5 possible, women = 1.6). The complexities of these issues were illuminated in the accounts of the interviewees.

Accounts of migration: material and professional considerations

Two issues dominated the physicians' views of migration: the low salaries of physicians and the difficulties in settling in a new country and, once settled, the difficulty in returning to their country. The two issues were given different emphasis in the accounts of paediatricians and surgeons. For the paediatricians, the material rewards of medical work in another country were the primary attraction for leaving. In general, the lack of dramatic change in the Lithuanian healthcare system – with few positive effects from a marketisation of healthcare and the remains of a devalued profession from the old state-ruled system – was viewed as impairing the work conditions for primary care physicians. As a university-related, middle-aged male paediatrician noted:

> 'And in general for sure, if the situation like this continues and the prospects do not change, very many and very good physicians [will leave]. Now, those who are young, who are most gifted, well, they leave – especially nursing staff, by the thousands. During the last week, two medical workers – one from the reception – left. Relatives of mine, some of them have left. Among my colleagues, maybe eight or nine left during the last two years. Well, I do not know the statistics, but that's how it is. … I also have considered like this: although for me it's not that bad here, I mean, I like my job here, but for sure it doesn't correspond to my qualifications. It is hard to subsist [on my current salary].' (Male paediatrician, #7)

Another older female paediatrician commented on the attractions of the professional conditions abroad:

> "So I'm very upset and it's enormously sad for me to see that they [my medical students] are leaving … many have already left or gone into the wholesale pharmaceutical business, many gifted young paediatricians, who could later succeed us in our positions. But they are leaving for a single reason. They are not leaving because of big ideas or professional improvement; they are leaving because of money. Money is the only reason.' (Female paediatrician, #34)

Table 14.2: Means and standard deviations for ICO and EO: physicians by gender and specialty

	Total		
	Total	Men	Women
Total (N/%)	137 100%	54 39%	83 61%
ICO: I have very good opportunities to leave for foreign countries to develop			
my professional career	2.48 (1.16)	2.96 (1.11)	2.18***a (1.10)
EO: I could leave for another country without any problems	3.03 (1.11)	3.25 (1.07)	2.89 (1.12)
	Paediatrics		
	Subtotal	Men	Women
Subtotalx (n/%)	43 31%	4 9%	39 91%
ICO: I have very good opportunities to leave for foreign countries to develop			
my professional career	2.12 (1.00)	2.75 (0.96)	2.05 (1.00)
EO: I could leave for another country without any problems	2.83 (1.08)	3.00 (0.82)	2.82 (1.11)
	Surgery		
	Subtotal	Men	Women
Subtotalx (n/%)	21 15%	16 76%	5 24%
ICO: I have very good opportunities to leave for foreign countries to develop			
my professional career	2.39 (1.29)	2.69 (1.32)	1.60 (0.89)
EO: I could leave for another country without any problems	3.05 (1.15)	3.13 (1.19)	2.80 (1.10)

Table 14.2: Means and standard deviations for ICO and EO: physicians by gender and specialty (continued)

	General practice		
	Subtotal	Men	Women
Subtotal[x] (n/%)	23 17%	9 39%	14 61%
ICO: I have very good opportunities to leave for foreign countries to develop my professional career	2.29 (1.19)	2.88 (1.25)	1.92 (1.04)
EO: I could leave for another country without any problems	2.91 (0.90)	3.22 (1.09)	2.71 (0.73)
	Other[xx]		
	Subtotal	Men	Women
Subtotal[x] (n/%)	47 34%	23 49%	24 51%
ICO: I have very good opportunities to leave for foreign countries to develop my professional career	2.94**b,d (1.15)	3.22 (1.00)	2.67 (1.24)
EO: I could leave for another country without any problems	3.28 (1.21)	3.39 (1.08)	3.17 (1.34)

Notes: Standard deviations are given in parentheses; means between men's and women's evaluations are statistically different at: *** 0.001 level (2-tailed); ** 0.01 level (2-tailed); * 0.05 level (2-tailed).

a - Statistically different means between men's and women's responses.
b - Statistically different means between paediatricians' and others' responses.
c - Statistically different means between surgeons' and others' responses.
d - Statistically different means between GPs' and others' responses.

x - Percentages for *subtotals* were calculated then 100% (N=137) for whole group in specialty and then 100% (n=) in particular specialties for men's and women's groups separately.

xx - In this category: *Men:* 4 in otolaryngology, 3 in nephrology and in orthopaedics, 2 in odontology, urology, neurology and radiotherapy and 1 in anaesthesiology, cardiology, clinical radiology, psychiatry and rheumatology; *Women:* 6 in nephrology, 4 in cardiology, 2 in clinical psychology and 1 in odontology, otolaryngology, rheumatology, anaesthesiology, infectious diseases, kinaesthesia, orthopaedics, psychotherapy, pulmonology and logopaedics.

There is also active recruitment going on from representatives of the international medical community. A male paediatrician said:

> 'Just a week ago, my last offer was to go to America, to a children's hospital in Boston. And the professor came here, and he said they need me there, and there are career possibilities. But they gave me just few hours to consider the offer and I told them no. So, that was my answer. It was one of the best offers – it was very specific, very particular, very real.' (Male paediatrician, #27)

Most paediatricians suggest that the low salaries of physicians compared to salaries of other workers is the primary motive for leaving. An older female paediatrician said:

> 'I would earn more. You understand, my salary is really small. There is nothing to hide and nothing to talk about, but it's that way. The salary is – I am ashamed to say how small my salary is [laughing]. I was taking care of the kids of my school friend and [she] said, well, you shouldn't stand for that, and what's your salary in roubles? After I told her, she said, Jesus Christ, my cleaning staff makes twice that. So I said, please take me on, I will work for you, and she said, oh, I can't do that, I wouldn't be comfortable with it.' (Female paediatrician, #8)

The material rewards for leaving are also attracting surgeons. As a middle-aged male surgeon noted:

> 'I think the situation is getting worse. As I have said, people are leaving. There will be a problem soon with the doctors, with the specialists. When someone leaves, someone else has to fill the position. But there is nobody who could do that. There are no others, because all the young physicians, all of them [have left] already, all the residents. I have asked them. All of them have their position there already – somewhere, something. They are leaving already. They are not even trying to get a position here. And this is the problem.' (Male surgeon, #9)

The second issue emphasised in the interviews is the difficulty in fitting into the new professional environment abroad and then again when returning to Lithuania with qualifications that are not necessarily needed and rewarded in the current structure of the profession and the healthcare system. This issue was highlighted in the female surgeons' accounts. As a young, female surgeon, who was hesitant to leave, reflected:

> 'Why should I? I have a job, this job here. I can tell you, all my achievements are due to my hard work. Why should I escape? There,

I won't be the same person as.... Well, there, probably, I won't be a
doctor.... Maybe you can pass an examination, you can make your
way up as a professional. Another thing is my parents are here, all my
relatives and friends. I would not like to leave. I am that kind of person.
I am close to my friends, relatives. I am related to this place. If I have
to leave, I would be hurt.' (Female surgeon, #2)

The difficulty in transferring from a job as a surgeon in different systems is
noted in several of the surgeons' accounts. For example, a young female surgeon
observed:

'Now it is very, very, very hard. If I leave, then imagine, for me, it would
mean that I would still have 10 years of active professional activity. So,
I would need to work very, very hard for 10 years before retirement.
What would be the meaning of that? When you come back, you have
to build your own private practice here. Nobody will be waiting for
you here. I can imagine that you will not be welcomed here with your
new qualifications, not in state institutions, maybe in private [practice].'
(Female surgeon, #5)

This view is echoed in another female surgeon's account:

'But I know that if you leave, there is nothing to come back for, because
you don't find anything after you here. I mean, an empty place remains
[when one leaves].... And nothing remains of what you were doing
– the ties are broken. It's very hard to start over. It takes many years to
restore your professional position.... The longer you work, the less
they are waiting for you here. There will be others who will have
taken your niche. They will not necessarily be doing what you did.
They will operate in some other way. But they will not at all like you
to come [back]. I think that's not only in Lithuania, that's all over the
world. There's a natural competition. Who will be waiting for you
here?' (Female surgeon, #1)

The main reported motivation for a career abroad in this study was a better income.
This issue was more often mentioned in the paediatricians' accounts than in the
surgeons', but neither saw professionalism or professional autonomy as a reason for
moving. The Lithuanian physicians are members of a profession who are used to
an employed status. In no account was the devalued status linked to the 'feminised'
character of the profession, but rather to the weak market condition vis-à-vis
other workers. For the surgeons, migration was not unconditionally valorised as
a future prospect. An intended move was evaluated against the more complex
division of labour and use of new medical technology abroad, a circumstance that

not only would devalue their skills even further if they migrated, but also render their newly acquired skills unusable if they were to return to Lithuania.

Conclusion

This study explored attitudes about career options, market conditions and changing governance among physicians practising in Lithuania. The survey results showed marked gender and specialty differences in the perceived possibilities of migrating and the opportunities for developing a career abroad. Men evaluated their options for leaving in more positive terms than did women, and also their opportunities for developing their professional career abroad. Similarly, surgeons were more optimistic about leaving and about a career abroad than were paediatricians. Nevertheless, in the interviews, the accounts were more nuanced.

For the paediatricians, the reason for migration was mainly defined in economic terms, while the surgeons were hesitant about whether they would fit into the structure of work abroad. In this regard, the surgeons were more realistic about their market position abroad than the paediatricians. On the other hand, the paediatricians might have had more confidence in the future positive effects of marketisation for their work conditions in their own country than the surgeons, whose field is rapidly declining because of the increasing use of laparoscopic technology in routine surgery (Zetka, 2003). Female surgeons foresaw these changes in their work and the difficulties in migrating more clearly than did male surgeons, who were more optimistic about their future work conditions.

The gendered and specialty-related views on migration and professional career options indicate their salience in societies in transition like Lithuania. Reprofessionalisation calls for within-state professional unity to advance a joint professional project, while international professional mobility is part of the scientific advances taking place in medical science and biotechnology. Professional career paths are today tied more to international scientific advances in the field than simply to within-state professional activities (Evetts, 1999; Leicht and Fennell, 2001). Reprofessionalisation and professional career mobility of physicians have gendered implications in post-Soviet societies because of the high proportion of women in the medical profession. The two developments need to be further explored in future research on the medical profession in these societies.

References

Abbott, A. (1988) *The system of professions: An essay on the division of expert labor*, Chicago, IL: University of Chicago Press.

Astor, A., Akthar, T., Matallana, M.A., Muthuswamy, V., Olowy, F.A., Tallo, V. and Lie, R.K. (2005) 'Physician migration: view from professionals in Columbia, Nigeria, India, Pakistan and the Philippines', *Social Science and Medicine*, vol 61, pp 2492-500.

Barr, D. and Boyle, E.H. (2001) 'Gender and professional purity: explaining formal and informal work rewards for physicians in Estonia', *Gender and Society*, vol 15, pp 29-54.

Barr, D.A. (1995) 'The professional structure of Soviet medical care: the relationship between personal characteristics, medical education and occupational setting for Estonian physicians', *American Journal of Public Health*, vol 85, pp 373-8.

Budani, D. (2005) 'Review of *Immigrant women tell their stories* by Roni Berger', *Gender and Society*, vol 19, p 710.

Charles, M. and Grusky, D.B. (2004) *Occupational ghettos: The worldwide segregation of women and men*, Stanford, CA: Stanford University Press.

Charmaz, K. (2006) *Constructing grounded theory: A practical guide through qualitative analysis*, Thousand Oaks, CA: Sage Publications.

Evetts, J. (1999) 'Professional identities: state and international dynamics in engineering', in I. Hellberg, M. Saks and C. Benoit (eds) *Professional identities in transition: Cross-cultural dimensions*, Södertälje: Almqvist & Wiksell International, pp 13-25.

Field, M. (1957) *Doctor and patient in Soviet Russia*, Cambridge, MA: Harvard University Press.

Field, M. (1967) *Soviet socialized medicine: An introduction*, New York: The Free Press.

Field, M. (1991) 'The hybrid profession: Soviet medicine', in A. Jones (ed) *Professions and the state: Expertise and autonomy in the Soviet Union and Eastern Europe*, Philadelphia, PA: Temple University, pp 43-62.

Freidson, E. (2001) *Professionalism: The third logic*, Chicago, IL: University of Chicago Press.

Gaižauskienė, A., Grabauskas, V., Kučinskienė, Z., Lovkytė, L., Vaitkienė, R., Paidaiga, Ž., Paskevičius, L., Petkevičius, R., Pūras, D., Reamy, J., Sinicienė, V. and Stankūnas, M. (2002) *Lietuvos gydytojų skaičiaus raida ir planavimas 1990-2015 metais*, ALF projekto 'Sveikatos žmogiškųjų išteklių raida ir planavimas Lietuvoje' ataskaita, Vilnius: Atviros Lietuvos Fondas, www.politika.osf.lt/visuomenes_sveikata/dokumentai/GSP_leidinys.pdf (in English: www.politika.osf.lt/public_health/documents/LGP_leidinys_engl.pdf)

Glaser, B.G. and Strauss, A.L. (1967) *The discovery of grounded theory*, Chicago, IL: Aldine de Gruyter.

Gliosaitė, K. (2004) 'Ekonomini emigracijos motyvų ir pasekmių vertinimas', seminario *'Šiuolaikinė lietuvių emigracija: Praradimai ir laimėjimai'* (seminar *Recent emigration of Lithuanians: Losses and Gains*), Vytauto Didžiojo Universiteyas, Kaunas, 2 December, www.civitas.lt/files/Konferencija_Emigracija_04_12_02_pranesimai.pdf

Guibernau, M. and Rex, J. (1997) *The ethnicity: Nationalism, multiculturalism, and migration*, Cambridge: Polity Press.

Hagopian, A., Ofosu, A., Fatusi, A., Biritwum, R., Essel, A., Hart, L.G. and Watts, C. (2005) 'The flight of physicians from West Africa: views of African physicians and implications for policy', *Social Science and Medicine*, vol 61, pp 1750-60.

Harrison, M. (1998) 'Female physicians in Mexico: migration and mobility in the life course', *Social Science and Medicine*, vol 47, pp 455-68.

Jones, A. (ed) (1991) *Professions and the state: Expertise and autonomy in the Soviet Union and Eastern Europe*, Philadelphia, PA: Temple University Press.

Leicht, K.T. and Fennell, M.L. (2001) *Professional work: A sociological approach*, Malden, MA: Blackwell.

Marcinkevičienė, R. (2004) 'Emigracija spaudoje: požiūrio atspindys ar formavimas', seminario *Šiuolaikinė lietuvių emigracija: Praradimai ir laimėjimai* (seminar *Recent emigration of Lithuanians: Losses and Gains*), Vytauto Didžiojo Universiteyas, Kaunas, 2 December, www.civitas.lt/files/Konferencija_Emigracija_04_12_02_pranesimai.pdf

Ministry of Health of Republic of Lithuania (2000) *Data of physician license registry*, Report No. 2000-03-18-48/8, Vilnius: Ministry of Health of Republic of Lithuania.

Osinsky, P. and Mueller, C.W. (2004) 'Professional commitment of Russian provincial specialists', *Work and Occupations*, vol 31, no 2, pp 193-224.

Raghuram, P. (2004) 'Migration, gender, and the IT sector: interesting debates', *Women's Studies International Forum*, vol 27, pp 163-76.

Riska, E. (2001a) *Medical careers and feminist agendas: American, Scandinavian and Russian women physicians*, New York: Aldine de Gruyter.

Riska, E. (2001b) 'Towards gender balance: but will women physicians have an impact on medicine?', *Social Science and Medicine*, vol 52, pp 179-87.

Rivkin-Fish, M. (2005) *Women's health in post-Soviet Russia: The politics of intervention*, Bloomington, IN: Indiana University Press.

Ryan, L. (2005) 'Questions of migration: geographical and transnational mobility in the twenty-first century', *Sociology*, vol 39, no 2, pp 381-8.

Ryan, M. (1989) *Doctors and the state in Soviet Union*, London: Macmillan.

Stankønienë, V. (ed) (1996) *Mobility of scientists in Lithuania: Internal and external brain drain*, Vilnius: STI.

Stankunas, M., Lovkyte, L. and Padaiga, Ž. (2004) 'The survey of Lithuanian physicians and medical residents regarding possible migration to the European Union (article in Lithuanian)', *Medicina*, vol 40, no 1, pp 68-74.

Stevens, F. (2005) 'The convergence and divergence of modern health care systems', in W.C. Cockerham (ed) *The Blackwell companion to medical sociology*, Oxford: Blackwell, pp 159-76.

Twigg, J.L. (2000) 'Unfilled hopes: the struggle to reform Russian health care and its financing', in M.G. Field and J.L. Twigg (eds) *Russia's torn safety nets: Health and social welfare during the transition*, New York: St. Martin's Press, pp 43-64.

WHO (World Health Organization) (1996) *Health care systems in transition: Lithuania*, Copenhagen: WHO Regional Office for Europe.

Zetka Jr., J.R. (2003) *Surgeons and the scope*, Ithaca, NY: Cornell University Press.

Health policy and workforce dynamics: the future

Ellen Kuhlmann and Mike Saks

This book has attempted to open up new perspectives in the topical health policy debate on professional governance that has become increasingly widely discussed in academic, policy and practice contexts. In this respect, we have argued for the need to link public policy and governance in healthcare to the study of professions. It has been our intention to add greater sophistication to, and provide more empirical evidence on, the complex 'colonising' debate on changing models of governance – currently biased towards both Anglo-American approaches and medical governance – instead of offering another 'quick fix' to a health policy debate overshadowed by normative assumptions on 'what works'. Greater sensitivity to national and cultural contexts and the varieties of professional groups and interests involved in healthcare may help us to better understand the translation of policies into practice and back again – the 'how' of the changes associated with new health policies.

The research contained in this volume brings into view a diverse and fluid workforce – that includes new professional groups and new forms of professionalism – which is responding to the changing demands on healthcare. It also puts the spotlight on the multiple challenges arising from integration and collaboration that have too often been overlooked in the policy debate. Focusing on the key themes of policy and workforce change, the book looks across countries and professional groups, mapping out key trends.

We now review the main findings across the chapters through the lens of the topics outlined in the Introduction and highlight the novel contribution the book makes to the debate over how to govern health professions. We begin by discussing the significance of the nation state as a navigator and the demand for institutional regulation across the various health professional groups, and how this is connected to new forms of professionalism. This is followed by tracing the translation of new forms of governance into professional development and the reconfiguration of boundaries, highlighting opportunities as well as new risks. The dynamics of de-regulation and the demands for re-regulation are also considered with regard to a mobile workforce, including different challenges, such as the gendered flexibilisation of work arrangements and migration tracks. We conclude by highlighting some issues regarding the future governance of a diverse international healthcare workforce.

Changing policies, changing professions: the nation state as a navigator

The comparison of medical governance in a wide range of healthcare systems by Allsop and Jones in Chapter One underlines the growing significance of network-based, partnership regulation that has been important in the transformation of professional self-regulation. This includes, for instance, new forms of assessment and control that are now more often exercised through public bodies, the establishment of various forms of continuing education, and dealing with poor practice. It also encompasses in a number of countries a broader range of health professions operating within legislative frameworks with greater emphasis on patient safety.

Similar trends are evident in the changing governance of medical providers and, as Burau and Vrangbæk conclude from a comparison of European health systems in Chapter Two, countries only vary in the relative balance of different forms of such governance. Using more 'fine-tuned' analysis, the authors are able to specify the composition of governance practices in different countries and to explore how national regulatory frameworks shape the opportunities for tighter regulation. The findings in these chapters therefore seem to confirm some degree of convergence of both health systems and the challenges to professional self-regulation; at the same time, the comparison of international and European directions in the changing governance of healthcare reveals developments that may contradict this idea and call for new approaches to understanding health policy.

The state–professions relationship revisited

One key conclusion drawn from the research outlined in this book is the significance of national pathways of transformation that continue to shape opportunity structures for the medical profession – which in many cases illustrates the institutional embeddedness of medical power. Another conclusion is that hierarchical governance persists alongside other forms of governance – and may even be reinforced by new models of network-based governance. A third conclusion highlights the connectivity of policy changes and changes in the professions. In this respect, tighter regulation and governmental and public intervention in the self-regulatory capacities of the medical profession do not necessarily cause overt conflict with professional interests. This may partly be a result of the privileged position that doctors enjoy in the health system. It also suggests, however, that the loss of power of the medical profession, or parts of the profession, in a single country may be replaced by new ways of exercising power (Harrison and McDonald, 2003; Salter, 2007). This increasingly includes the flows of power of medical professionalism operating as an international force (Kuhlmann and Burau, forthcoming). Furthermore, policy goals may be supported by developments in the professions and vice versa, although this does not necessarily mean the end of 'turf battles'.

These trends point to the significance of the state–professions relationship as a key to better understanding the 'how' of policy changes. It directs our attention to topical issues in the sociology of professions: namely the role of the state (Johnson et al, 1995), the ethics of professional self-regulation (Allsop and Saks, 2002), and the relationship between the 'private interest government' (Moran, 1999) and the 'altruistic mission' of professionalism to serve what is defined as the 'public interest' (Saks, 1995). Professions are expected to be accountable to both governments and citizens. Consequently, they may counteract the state and the market as a 'third logic' (Freidson, 2001), and also act in accordance with political and market interests in health and other areas. They may be champions of the 'people', especially patients, and also exercise their own private interests. The dualism and the tensions embedded in professionalism continue to persist in new forms of professional governance.

The linkage between policy changes and professional development is further explored in this book by using national configurations of professional governance and new professional groups as case studies. Professionalism embodies a number of regulatory mechanisms that are essential for the functioning of health systems – and societies at large. Stacey (1992), drawing on the General Medical Council and the National Health Service (NHS) in Britain, has highlighted the capacity of self-regulatory professions to 'buffer' social conflict. The approach to professions as mediators between governments and citizens as set out by Kuhlmann in Chapter Three of this volume may therefore be helpful in uncovering the intersections of professionalism and changing governance practices.

One important area where these intersections may challenge health policy is in building trust in healthcare. There is an increasing concern over the potentially adverse effects of managerialist regimes on trust relations, which are often used to foster the normative claims of the medical profession against demands for greater public control and transparency of services. The more complex framework for researching trust relations in healthcare highlighted in Chapter Four by Calnan and Rowe reveals transformations, but in uneven ways: health reform and changing governance embody both risk and opportunity for professionals, patients and managers. The classic model of 'embodied' trust – 'Trust me, I'm a doctor' – is no longer convincing, while at the same time, public trust in doctors remains high. Furthermore, improved provision of, and access to, information provides new opportunities for patients to build 'informed' trust in providers (see Allsop, 2006; Kuhlmann, 2006; Schee et al, 2007). These developments point to changes in the concepts of both trust and professionalism. While the debate on a decline of trust in healthcare focuses on the citizens'/patients' perspective, the approach introduced by Calnan and Rowe also underlines the significance of professional relationships, which may be a facilitator or inhibitor of collaborative care. The fruitfulness of an approach based on trust as 'organiser' of interprofessional relationships is confirmed by the empirical research into different professional groups and countries presented in this volume, to which we shall return later.

A new professionalism in the making?

Evidence for emerging new forms of professionalism, which amalgamate managerialist approaches with professional action and agency, is reported from a number of different health systems, such as Australia and Germany. This suggests that new health policies – including changing macro-level institutional regulation and policy frameworks, as well as meso-level governance and organisational conditions – do provide opportunities for professions to exercise power and promote their interests in the changing world of governance. This can be reassuring to professions, as in the case of the medical profession in Germany with a configuration of governance that excludes players other than the medical profession, as highlighted in Chapter Three. It can also facilitate the professionalisation of new groups, as in the case of Australian allied health professionals working in hospitals that Boyce outlines in Chapter Five, where a wide range of professional groups is now included in the regulatory frameworks and the organisation of care. This brings into focus the specific configuration of the state–professions relationship that can foster or limit the professionalisation of new groups (Saks, 2003; Bourgeault, 2006).

Studies on new forms of professionalism also highlight the options for, and barriers to, the emergence of more inclusive forms of professionalism that are now typically sought within the national regulatory frameworks of healthcare systems. As noted in Chapter Three, the German system may lack regulatory bodies for the majority of the health workforce not acknowledged as professions, but provides some evidence of the development of a more inclusive professionalism, albeit one that varies between groups. In consequence, the different professional groups cannot use the opportunities provided by new health policies as effectively as the medical profession, because they lack the power to take collective action and to forge an identity. In contrast, in the Australian case set out in Chapter Five, with more advanced regulation of the entire health workforce, more inclusive forms of professionalism are emerging in the allied health professions; as Boyce observes, this is closely linked to organisational restructuring and includes new resources for developing 'lateral' collective professional identities as 'allied health professions'. The following section further explores the ties and tensions between regulatory frameworks, new policies and professional action and agency, and how they may enable greater collaboration between professional groups.

Professional collaboration: policy goal and policy challenge

The making of a more integrated and collaborative health workforce is a key policy goal in many countries. The exclusionary tactics of the medical profession are commonly perceived as the main barrier to more integrated caring models and professional collaboration. As a consequence, both policy debate and research have focused on social exclusion and the 'boundary work' of the medical profession, often using nursing and the gendered order of the medical profession as examples (see, for instance, Witz, 1992). However, with the emergence of a wide range of new professional projects, together with changing health policies and the shifting organisation of healthcare, there are ever more boundaries in the health workforce to be contested, transformed or removed. Added to this, professionalism may facilitate occupational change, but plays out differently in established and new professional groups, as Evetts (2006) has highlighted. It is argued here that we need to look in more detail at emerging professional groups and the varieties of professionalism rather than simply focusing on the exclusionary tactics of the medical profession.

Research indicates that there has been a general trend towards more inclusive forms of professionalism in all professional groups – including medicine – although with considerable variation in the shifts and permeability of professional boundaries (Dahl, 2005; Jones and Green, 2006; McKee et al, 2006; Nancarrow and Borthwick, 2006). To this end, new health policies create dynamics in the health workforce, but across countries the future of a collaborative workforce remains uncertain. The studies included in this book bring into focus a wide range of enabling conditions as well as 'blockers' of integration, and illustrate that boundary work is not limited to the medical profession.

As Bourgeault and Darling note in Chapter Six, the contestation of professional boundaries was observed in the profession of midwifery in Canada – and was also apparent, as Iarskaia-Smirnova and Romanov highlight in Chapter Nine, among providers of complementary and alternative medicine (CAM) in Russia. These two examples are especially interesting because both professional groups claim to have a more 'holistic' and inclusive therapeutic approach. However, the case studies reveal that this does not easily translate into removing boundaries when it comes to work relations and professional interests (see also Saks, 2003). Nonetheless, there is some evidence from the studies presented that the driving force towards collaboration may be stronger in professional groups other than medicine – as is further underlined by nurses in Slovenia as indicated by Pahor in Chapter Seven of this volume.

The studies in this book suggest that no single factor can account for the creation of a collaborative health workforce, and no single professional group can be identified as a 'change agent'. Instead, opportunities for, and barriers to, collaboration exist in all countries. The conceptual model of the complex range of factors influencing collaborative care articulated by Bourgeault and Darling covers the macro, meso and micro level, such as funding regimes, the mix of providers in the community and also pre-existing interprofessional relationships. Despite these general conclusions, a number of more specific factors furthering professional collaboration can be identified from the studies in this collection. These include hierarchical forms of governance – such as regulatory bodies, registers and other forms of institutional regulation – as well as culture and more decentralised and managerialist models of governance characteristic of the new public management (NPM).

Regulating the healthcare workforce: new opportunity structures

Tighter institutional regulation of a broad range of health professional groups can nonetheless be viewed as the strongest single factor that facilitates both a more inclusive health workforce and the professionalisation of new groups. This is indicated most clearly in the case of health support workers and CAM practitioners in the UK, on which Saks focuses in Chapter Ten of this volume. Regulation impacts as a facilitator of occupational change where professional recognition has been built up, as highlighted by the allied health professions in Australia in Chapter Five and the relatively new profession of midwifery in Canada in Chapter Six. This may also be relevant in the Russian case outlined in Chapter Nine, where government action in regulating CAM practitioners has been extended, although not to the same extent as in the Anglo-Saxon countries. In the German case set out in Chapter Three, there is conversely a correlation between a lack of comprehensive regulation and low levels of professionalisation of the various health professional groups, including nursing, compared to other European countries.

There is also evidence for new opportunity structures embedded in comprehensive health workforce regulation across very different healthcare systems, spanning from the Anglo-Saxon national health systems and the corporatist-based German system to the transformation system in Russia. The argument is implicitly supported too by the finding of Burau and Vrangbæk in Chapter Two that hierarchical forms of governance remain strong in an era of decentralisation and network governance. However, government efforts to regulate the healthcare workforce may play out differently in different national contexts. As Saks notes in Chapter Ten, the drivers for regulating the healthcare workforce include economic incentives to reduce staffing costs – by, for instance, delegating work to lower-status professions, changing the skill mix and redistributing work – as well as the desire to improve the safety of the service user, and professional self-interests. The precise combination of drivers, players and interests involved in the establishment of new regulatory bodies may therefore vary greatly between countries, and existing power structures may be challenged in different ways, either provoking resistance or supportive action.

The research studies in this book therefore suggest that opportunity structures for collaboration derive from the specific configuration of macro-level regulation and meso- and micro-level conditions in the field. The examples of allied health professions in Australia and midwives in Canada highlight such opportunities. The coming together of drivers at all levels may consequently help us to predict new patterns of a more inclusive professionalism – based on 'lateral identities' – as well as more collaborative caring teams.

New public management and 'flexible' professionalism: the coming together of opportunity and risk

NPM is a cornerstone of new forms of governance and an umbrella term for a number of managerialist regulatory mechanisms aimed at bringing more efficiency into the healthcare sector, including improved user 'choice' and demand-led services. NPM includes the regulatory mechanisms governing economic life (Miller and Rose, 1990) and a discourse of modernisation linked to flexibility, individualisation and 'freedom of choice' (Johnson, 1995; Flynn, 2004). As such, NPM is a highly flexible governance practice that needs to be made more concrete in order to explore its impact in healthcare, and more specifically in the transformation of professionalism. NPM includes various rules and incentives for professional development, such as continuing education and monitoring the quality of services. It also supports 'flexible' professionalism. However, NPM does not provide a coherent strategy for improving collaboration between providers, although some organisations have introduced incentives for collaboration. In addition, it is not very adequately linked to macro-level regulatory frameworks.

Given the nature of NPM regimes, the studies presented here unsurprisingly reveal no consistent pattern of change. As mentioned previously in Chapter Five in relation to the Australian case of allied health professions, NPM provides opportunity structures for more inclusive forms of professionalism and identity. In a similar vein, new opportunities for auxiliary nursing in Finland are documented by Wrede in Chapter Eight of this book. However, at the same time, this example indicates that there can be potentially adverse effects on professionalism and the construction of professional identities. This is because the introduction of educational systems creating 'flexible' generalists in low-status segments of the health workforce and the dissolution of occupational boundaries as a result of organisational interests may mean that there is a lack of resources for collective identity and action, and consequent dissatisfaction of the workers involved. Indeed, these developments may even reinforce hierarchy and exclusionary strategies. Nonetheless, the low status of a professional group does not fully explain these developments. Dahle and Skogheim in Chapter Eleven describe similar problems in Norway among qualified nurses working in agency organisations.

The most important conclusions we can draw from research in this area in this volume is that, first, managerialist regimes embody both opportunity structures for a more inclusive professionalism and barriers to professional development in – mainly female – occupational groups; second, a more 'flexible' professionalism is not necessarily a more inclusive model, but may create new inequalities; and, third, managerialism and flexible professionalism both create new pressures for the management of risk and vulnerability. Consequently, managerialism and flexibility reinforce the significance of hierarchical intervention and tighter workforce regulation, especially of lower-status occupational groups more vulnerable to market forces and the exclusionary tactics of established professions. At a more general level, this finding mirrors the linkage between strong markets and strong states (see Freeman, 1998; Kuhlmann and Burau, forthcoming).

Hidden organisers of collaboration and boundary work: culture and trust

Culture has a considerable impact on the opportunities for collaboration. This is a relatively overlooked dimension in establishing the conditions for collaboration, although it is increasingly emphasised in governance theory and empirical research (see, for instance, Newman, 2001). Clarke (2005, p 19) highlights that Europe is already multiracial, multi-ethnic and multinational and underlines that 'an "Anglo-Saxon" European model of unity clearly lacks both empirical and political plausibility'. The loosening of boundaries within Europe, together with globalisation and migration, means that there is a growing need to take account of cultural diversity in healthcare. The concept of 'culture' itself is highly diverse and fluid – and, as such, a challenge, if not an obstacle to comparative research. As the research studies in this book indicate, though, however defined, cultural values impact on the willingness of professionals to collaborate.

In Chapter Seven, Pahor, drawing on comparative research into collaboration between doctors, nurses and nursing assistants in Slovenia, highlights that attitudes are shaped by a Roman Catholic culture in a society marked by the legacy of the centralised bureaucracy of the socialist era with strong contemporary patterns of individualism – leading to lower levels of generalised trust and collaboration. In this case, the particular configuration of cultural values may be a barrier, and Europeanisation together with international – 'Westernising' – directions in healthcare may foster greater collaboration between professionals. While culture remains an implicit factor in the Slovenian case, it can also be used more explicitly as 'social capital' to improve market power, as has been shown by Iarskaia-Smirnova and Romanov in relation to Russian CAM practitioners in Chapter Nine. Here, culture provides a resource for 'boundary work' against the medical profession. Culture may also further collaboration if it is based on shared values across professional groups or professionals and service users. One such example is the case of midwifery described in Chapter Six and, more generally, that of women's healthcare teams. However, shared values are not sustainable in promoting collaboration when there is competition between providers (Bourgeault and Mulvale, 2006) or conflict of interest between professionals and service users (Benoit, 1999).

Another factor impacting on collaboration in healthcare is trust. Evidence from different countries and professional groups suggests that the building of trustworthy relationships between different provider groups may engender more positive attitudes towards collaboration and enhance the willingness to collaborate. This was observed in the cases of collaboration between midwives and doctors in Canada in Chapter Six, the Slovenian nursing and medical profession in Chapter Seven and CAM practitioners and orthodox doctors in Russia in Chapter Nine. Here, it is important to recall the model of researching trust set out in this book by Calnan and Rowe in Chapter Four, which highlights the complex interplay of various players and conditions that shape the building of trust relations. Pahor in Chapter Seven has also shown that the willingness to build trust is shaped by cultural traditions, which in the Slovenian case may have had a negative impact. This example underlines the complexity of the transformations linked to international governance and converging nation states that cannot be explained by simply looking at health policy but need further investigation.

Reconfiguring a mobile health workforce: de-regulation and re-regulation

Changing health policies increasingly interface with labour market changes and changing patterns of individual arrangements relating to work, career and life, including the decision to migrate in order to improve life chances. The case studies in this book explore these developments from the perspective of the actors in various professional groups in the health workforce, spanning from doctors to nurses and newly emerging occupational groups 'in between' health and other sectors. Micro-level changes in the professions are linked to broader societal changes, such as the de-regulation of work, lifestyle changes and new demands on health, wellness and fitness, as well as migration. Apart from results specific to the case studies, the research in this collection points to a number of general conclusions that have important consequences for health policy and professional governance.

One of the strongest conclusions is the ongoing significance of gender as a regulatory mechanism in the healthcare sector (see also Davies, 2002; Annandale, 2005). Although formal barriers to women's participation in the professions have been removed and gender equality is now monitored in most countries, inequality continues to persist; it is embedded – and hidden – in new models of de-regulated and flexible work and the flows of mobility and migration. This is shown by Dahle and Skogheim in Chapter Eleven of this volume in relation to agency organisations in Norway that provide new opportunities for women to combine more flexibly their work and life situations, including caring responsibilities. At the same time, they also create new 'gender traps' for qualified nurses. The sexual division of healthcare labour therefore remains significant and may even be reinforced in the emerging group of less-qualified auxiliary nurses, as Wrede indicates in Chapter Eight. Both studies in different ways highlight that attempts to create a flexible workforce through changing health policies open up individual opportunities, but also have potentially negative effects on collective professional identity and action. Moreover, as Formadi notes in Chapter Twelve of this book, in a newly established occupational group that crosses the boundaries between the health and tourism sector and strives for professionalisation, gender arrangements – which nowadays tend to appear as 'flexible' work/life balance – shape occupational mobility and career pathways.

In Chapter Fourteen Riska and Novelskaite observe that gender, together with speciality, also matters in the medical profession in a transformation society like Lithuania as regards attitudes to migration and career options abroad. Here, men evaluated their options for leaving in more positive terms than women, including their opportunities for developing their professional career in another country. Viewed from the perspective of migrants, the case of foreign professionals in the Portuguese NHS studied by Ribeiro in Chapter Thirteen highlights that, as both nurses and doctors, women face a number of obstacles to occupational integration. In this case, gender and ethnicity merge together as new patterns of social inequality and create new lines of division within healthcare professions. This was especially true of the group of migrants four countries that are not member states of the European Union.

The findings from the studies in this book also point to new tensions between 'within-state professional activities' (Evetts, 1999) and the demands of international professional governance. For instance, the existence of foreign health professionals in the Portuguese NHS documented in Chapter Thirteen prevents the concept of professional self-regulation being used as a basis for the hegemonic claims of national players against the interests of an ethnically diverse workforce. This point is also illustrated in Chapter Eleven by the Norwegian caring system, which resolves staff shortages in less attractive areas through the substitution of native with minority group professionals. However, both examples indicate that economic pressures on reducing staffing costs may lead to an exploitation of migrants, who are more vulnerable to market forces and less able to voice their demands.

Furthermore, an ongoing migration flow from less wealthy transformation societies – like Lithuania – to economically stronger nations with welfare states may cause a shortage of highly qualified healthcare staff in the home country of migrants as highlighted in Chapter Fourteen. Migration flows of health professionals may therefore have negative consequences on the quality of care in poorer countries, thereby becoming a policy problem (see Buchan, 2006). These conclusions raise new questions about both the self-regulatory capacity of professions to serve the interests of a changing public and professionalism as a national project (see Moran, 2002).

The studies in this collection also bring into view new risks relating to the safety of patients and other service users. For instance, the agency nurses in Norway described in Chapter Eleven often lack adequate information on patients and organisational issues, while there are risks inherent in the fact that the foreign professionals in Portugal referred to in Chapter Thirteen often work overtime. The intersecting areas of health and tourism in Hungarian spas in Chapter Twelve, meanwhile, raise the question of whether existing regulatory mechanisms in healthcare stretch far enough to cover such new groups 'in between' health and other occupational fields. In this respect, the case study more generally points to new professional services in need of regulation, such as home care and various forms of counselling.

Governing a diverse international healthcare workforce

The chapters presented in this collection underline the broad range of evolving regulatory mechanisms and governance practices and their links to institutional, social and cultural change. As editors, we have highlighted the benefits of, and pressures for, tighter regulation across the entire healthcare sector, including new groups at the margins, and how they intersect with national configurations of governance practices that may advance or block more inclusive forms of professionalism. The chapters also spotlight new demands for transnational regulation and the management of diversity and equality. A complex picture of the various modes of governance and how they are shaped and reshaped by interest-driven strategies of the professions and other factors thereby emerges, which throws up new policy options.

Whether the changes indicate that a 'new' form of professionalism is developing – as, for example, a more 'democratic' pattern – or only that there is a gradual shift in balance towards more inclusive types of professionalism remains to be seen. No straightforward roads to collaboration and professionalisation, and no uniform model of the 'new professional' (Dent and Whitehead, 2002) can currently be identified. Instead, there is evidence for increasingly diverse forms of professionalism and different strategies of professionalisation that embody the potential for more inclusive professional action and identity and the reconfiguration of boundaries within and between professional groups.

We can conclude from the research contained in this volume that new health policies – from tighter institutional regulation and the development of more inclusive regulatory bodies to NPM regimes – shape, but do not fully allow us to predict, future pathways to collaboration. In consequence, the key policy goal of creating a more collaborative health workforce is a challenge to health policy itself. Davies (2003), in her study of the future health workforce in the British NHS, raises the question of how far the 'workforce revolution' is a desired, rather than an actual, outcome of health policies. The studies presented in this book generate further scepticism – while at the same time providing further evidence for change. They seem to confirm the observation by Freeman (2000) that healthcare systems do not act very systematically.

As this volume has highlighted, rethinking the development of a more inclusive regulatory framework for the governance of a diverse future health workforce is a major issue for health policy internationally. However, there is an overall lack of systematic policy vision on furthering a 'learning system' of coordination and collaboration, related in part to existing patterns of professionalism and medical dominance. If this policy deficit is to be addressed, additional work will need to be undertaken to meet the challenges of social inclusion arising from a 'mobile' society and 'flexible work'. Future research is needed to better understand, first, the persistence of social inequalities, especially those relating to gender and ethnicity/nationality and how they are connected; second, the new tensions between national professional governance and international demands, such as migration flows; and, third, the new risks to the safety of patients and the quality of care, including those services at the margins of healthcare.

References

Allsop, J. (2006) 'Regaining trust in medicine: professional strategies', *Current Sociology*, vol 54, pp 621-36.

Allsop, J. and Saks, M. (eds) (2002) *Regulating the health professions*, London: Sage Publications.

Annandale, E. (2005) 'Missing connections: medical sociology and feminism', *Medical Sociology News*, vol 31, no 3, pp 35-52.

Benoit, C. (1999) 'Midwifery and health policy: equity, workers' rights and consumer choice in Canada and Sweden', in I. Hellberg, M. Saks and C. Benoit (eds) *Professional identities in transition: Cross-cultural dimensions*, Göteborg: Almquist & Wiksell, pp 255-74.

Bourgeault, I.L. (2006) *Push! The struggle for midwifery in Ontario*, Montreal: McGill-Queen's University Press.

Bourgeault, I.L. and Mulvale, G. (2006) 'Collaborative health care teams in Canada and the U.S.: confronting the structural embeddedness of medical dominance', *Health Sociology Review*, vol 15, no 5, pp 481-95.

Buchan, J. (2006) 'Migration of health workers in Europe: policy problem or policy solution?', in C.-A. Dubois, M. McKee and E. Nolte (eds) *Human resources for health in Europe*, Milton Keynes: Open University Press, pp 41-62.

Clarke, J. (2005) 'Reconstituting Europe: governing a European people', in J. Newman (ed) *Remaking governance: People, politics and the public sphere*, Bristol: The Policy Press, pp 17-37.

Dahl, H.M. (2005) 'Re-imagining the (welfare) professional as a specialised generalist', *Knowledge, Work and Society*, vol 3, no 2, pp 19-39.

Davies, C. (2002) 'Registering a difference: changes in the regulation of nursing', in J. Allsop and M. Saks (eds) *Regulating the health professions*, London: Routledge, pp 94-107.

Davies, C. (2003) 'Introduction: a new workforce in the making?', in C. Davies (ed) *The future health workforce*, Houndmills: Palgrave, pp 1-13.

Dent, M. and Whitehead, S. (2002) 'Introduction: configuring the "new" professional', in M. Dent and S. Whitehead (eds) *Managing professional identities*, London: Routledge, pp 1-18.

Evetts, J. (1999) 'Professional identities: state and international dynamics in engineering', in I. Hellberg, M. Saks and C. Benoit (eds) *Professional identities in transition: Cross-cultural dimensions*, Södertälje: Almqvist & Wiksell International, pp 13-25.

Evetts, J. (2006) 'The sociology of professional groups: new directions', *Current Sociology*, vol 54, no 1, pp 133-43.

Flynn, R. (2004) 'Soft bureaucracy, governmentality and clinical governance: theoretical approaches to emergent policy', in A. Grey and S. Harrison (eds) *Medical governance: Theory and practice*, Milton Keynes: Open University Press, pp 11-26.

Freeman, R. (1998) 'The German model: the state and the market in health care', in W. Ranade (ed) *Markets and health care: A comparative analysis*, London: Longman, pp 179-93.

Freeman, R. (2000) *The politics of health in Europe*, Manchester: Manchester University Press.

Freidson, E. (2001) *Professionalism: The third logic*, Oxford: Polity Press.

Harrison, S. and McDonald, R. (2003) 'Science, consumerism and bureaucracy – new legitimations of medical professionalism', *International Journal of Public Sector Management*, vol 16, no 2, pp 110-21.

Johnson, T. (1995) 'Governmentality and the institutionalization of expertise', in T. Johnson, G. Larkin and M. Saks (eds) *Health professions and the state in Europe*, London: Routledge, pp 7-24.

Johnson, T., Larkin, G. and Saks, M. (eds) (1995) *Health professions and the state in Europe*, London: Routledge.

Jones, L. and Green, J. (2006) 'Shifting discourses of professionalism: a case study of general practitioners in the United Kingdom', *Sociology of Health and Illness*, vol 28, pp 927-50.

Kuhlmann, E. (2006) *Modernising health care: Reinventing professions, the state and the public*, Bristol: The Policy Press.

Kuhlmann, E. and Burau, V. (forthcoming) 'The "healthcare state" in transition: national and international contexts of changing professional governance', *European Societies*, Thematic Issue.

McKee, M., Dubois, C.-A. and Sibbard, B. (2006) 'Changing professional boundaries', in C.-A. Dubois, M. McKee and E. Nolte (eds) *Human resources for health in Europe*, Milton Keynes: Open University Press, pp 63-78.

Miller, P. and Rose, N. (1990) 'Governing economic life', *Economy and Society*, vol 19, no 1, pp 1-31.

Moran, M. (1999) *Governing the health care state*, Manchester: Manchester University Press.

Moran, M. (2002) 'The health professionals in international perspective', in J. Allsop and M. Saks (eds) *Regulating the health professions*, London: Sage Publications, pp 19-30.

Nancarrow, S. and Borthwick, A. (2006) 'Dynamic professional boundaries in the healthcare workforce', *Sociology of Health and Illness*, vol 27, pp 897-919.

Newman, J. (2001) *Modernising governance: New Labour, policy and governance*, London: Sage Publications.

Saks, M. (1995) *Professions and the public interest: Medical power, altruism and alternative medicine*, London: Routledge.

Saks, M. (2003) *Orthodox and alternative medicine: Politics, professionalization and health care*, London: Sage Publications.

Salter, B. (2007) 'Governing UK medical performance: a struggle for policy dominance', *Health Policy*, vol 82, pp 263-75.

Schee, E. van der, Braun, B., Calnan, M., Schnee, M. and Groenewegen, P.P. (2007) 'Public trust in health care: a comparison of Germany, the Netherlands, and England and Wales', *Health Policy*, vol 81, pp 56-67.

Stacey, M. (1992) *Regulating British medicine: The General Medical Council*, Chichester: Wiley.

Witz, A. (1992) *Professions and patriarchy*, London: Routledge.

Index

Note: Page numbers in *italic* refer to figures and tables.

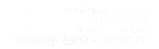

Lightning Source UK Ltd.
Milton Keynes UK
UKHW051013291118
332909UK00033B/886/P